WOMEN'S
EVERYDAY
HEALTH GUIDE

WOMEN'S EVERYDAY HEALTH GUIDE

BY
DR ROSEMARY LEONARD

BOXTREE

Advice to the Reader
Before following any medical or dietary advice contained in this book, it is recommended that you consult your doctor if you suffer from any health problems or special condition or are in any doubt as to its suitability.

B⊛XTREE

First published in 1996 by Boxtree,
an imprint of Macmillan Publishers Ltd,
25 Eccleston Place, London SW1W 9NF and Basingstoke.

Associated companies throughout the world.

1 3 5 7 9 10 8 6 4 2

ISBN 0 7522 0552 8

Designed by Blackjacks

Printed and bound in Great Britain by Cox & Wyman Ltd, Reading, Berkshire.

A CIP catalogue record for this book is available from the British Library

Foreword

It's very easy to take good health for granted. When you're used to being well, any illness can come as a nasty shock, and it's only natural to want an instant cure. But increasingly, the route back to tip-top condition needn't involve a time-consuming trip to your doctor's surgery. Many ills can be cured with simple, effective remedies available at either your local chemist, or even supermarket!

Not only that, but with just a little care and attention, and a few adjustments to your diet and lifestyle, many illnesses, including serious ones such as cancer and heart disease, can be prevented.

Through my experience working as a GP in a busy practice, I know that many women have unique health problems that cannot always be dealt with adequately in a standard seven-minute consultation. The aim of this book is to give both background information and practical advice about self-help. The emphasis is on conventional treatments, but well-tried and tested complementary therapies are included as well. It also explains when you should seek medical expertise – and the types of treatment you can expect to receive. There is extra detail on the topics that are especially important to women, such as breasts, contraception, and fertility. Inevitably, in a book of this size, it's just not possible to cover every single ailment, but the ones for women are all here. The one topic that is missing is pregnancy – but that's because I feel it deserves a whole book in its own right!

The book is laid out in alphabetical order. If you need additional information, I've included a list of useful organizations at the back.

ABORTION (OR TERMINATION)

This used to apply to any baby lost in the early stages of pregnancy, but now the term is mainly used to describe a woman's choice to terminate a pregnancy. This can be for personal reasons, such as when the pregnancy is unwanted, or medical reasons, such as when a much-wanted baby is found to be abnormal in some way.

Choosing to terminate a pregnancy is never easy, no matter what the circumstances, and it should never be a hurried decision. All women considering an abortion should make sure they talk it through thoroughly, ideally with the baby's father, as well as a health care professional, such as a GP or counsellor. Many good abortion clinics now routinely offer counselling to all women.

In this country, abortion can be performed legally up to the twenty-fourth week of pregnancy. Two doctors must agree that the procedure is justified for one of five reasons. These include not only whether the baby is likely to be severely handicapped, but also if the mother's physical or mental health is likely to be badly affected by the pregnancy. There is also another clause that allows the doctors to take into consideration the health of any of the mother's existing children.

Arranging an abortion

This section applies to women who have an unwanted pregnancy. Women who are found to have an abnormal baby are usually cared for automatically by either their GP or obstetrician. Abortions are available on the NHS, but the type of service provided can vary enormously in different parts of the country. Private abortions are also readily available country-wide, usually with minimal waiting times.

With abortions, speed counts. If you miss a period, do a pregnancy test without delay. This will give you the maximum amount of time to consider what you want to do. If you want a free abortion on the NHS, you'll need a referral letter from either your GP, or the doctor at your local family planning clinic.

Alternatively, you can contact a private clinic directly (they are listed in the telephone directory). However, it's essential that you go to one that provides a good, reliable service. Your GP should be happy to give you advice about this.

Private costs vary between clinics and according to the type of method used. Costs go up after twelve weeks, and again after fifteen weeks. Charity-based clinics, such as The British Pregnancy Advisory Service and Marie Stopes clinics, are generally cheaper than a private hospital with a private gynaecologist.

An abortion up to twelve weeks, in a charity based clinic, usually costs in the region of £250–300 (1996 prices).

What's involved?
There are three different types of abortion.

❶ A medical abortion can be done up until the end of the ninth week of pregnancy (sixty-three days from the first day of your last period). First, three pills containing the hormone mifepristone are taken by mouth. Two days later, a prostoglandin pessary is put in the vagina, and this normally induces a complete miscarriage within six hours. You stay at the hospital during this time, until the bleeding has died down. Many women experience quite severe cramps, but these can be eased by painkillers, which the hospital staff should provide. The majority of women are able to go home the same day. Occasionally however, the womb does not empty completely, and a D and C operation (see page 51), and an overnight hospital stay, is required to prevent excessive bleeding.

❷ The suction method is used for the vast majority of terminations, and is suitable for pregnancies up to twelve weeks (dated from the first day of the last period). Under either a local or a general anaesthetic, the neck of the womb is gently stretched (or dilated), and the content sucked out using a powerful vacuum. Women having this done under a local anaesthetic may find the sound of this quite distressing, but the whole procedure only takes about five minutes. It's normal to go home the same day. It's also normal to feel some cramps afterwards, but bleeding should be light.

❸ After twelve weeks, the womb has to be emptied using instruments, rather than suction. This requires a general anaesthetic, and one or two days in hospital. Many doctors find performing this type of later abortion quite distressing, and for this reason they are difficult to obtain on the NHS, unless the baby is deformed.

A

What are the risks?
Though the vast majority of abortions are quite straightforward, complications do occur, and can affect your future fertility. The most common are:
➤ incomplete emptying of the contents of the womb, leading to pain and heavy bleeding
➤ infection of the womb lining, which may spread up to the fallopian tubes, causing severe pelvic inflammation with scarring. An infection may occur on its own, but is more likely after the first example above.

Any women experiencing severe pain, heavy bleeding, the passage of clots, or a high temperature after an abortion should see a doctor straight away. Prompt treatment with antibiotics may help to safeguard your future fertility.

Afterwards
Use towels, not tampons, and avoid having sex until the bleeding has stopped. The combination of the mental strain, an operation and plummeting hormone levels mean that it's normal to feel upset, tired, drained and depressed after a termination, even if you have an underlying sense of relief. It's best to have a week off work, with plenty of rest. Having an abortion can have a huge impact on your emotions, and you need to give these time to recover.

ACNE
Though acne is often regarded as a teenage affliction, women of all ages can be affected.

In classic acne, excess sebum production, together with increased numbers of the bacteria on the skin surface, leads to blocked pores, which are visible as white heads and black heads. These often become inflamed, forming pustules or spots. In more serious cases, small abscesses may form, which can be very painful.

Acne should never be ignored. Apart from its unsightly cosmetic appearance, large spots can cause permanent scars. In older women, localized redness and spots across the nose and cheeks may be due to rosacea (see page 150). In some women, acne may be one of the symptoms, along with irregular periods and a tendency to hairiness, of polycystic ovarian syndrome (see page 144).

Self-help
➤ Keep your skin scrupulously clean, and keep infection at bay by

8

washing twice a day. Anti-bacterial skin washes are best, but these can cause allergic reactions.

➤ Apply a cream containing benzyl peroxide once or twice a day to affected areas. The cream can cause redness and dryness – start with a 5 percent strength, and work up to 10 percent if necessary.

➤ Even if you feel you need some camouflage, avoid wearing a heavy, oil-based foundation that will clog your pores even more. Use a lighter, non-comegic base instead (i.e. one that won't clog pores).

➤ On the affected areas use skin products designed for oily skin. This may mean having two different sets on the go – one for drier areas, such as around your eyes, and another for the greasy, spot-prone T-zone.

➤ Blackheads can be gently squeezed (after a hot bath is best), but never squeeze spots. It only spreads the inflammation and makes them look (and feel) worse then ever.

➤ Eat a healthy diet with plenty of fresh fruit and vegetables. Eating lots of greasy food and chocolate may make your acne worse, and neither are good for your general health.

Help from your doctor

➤ Antibiotics, particularly tetracyclines and erythromycin, can be very effective treatment, but they're not an instant cure. At least threee months treatment is required for any noticeable effect. They're available either as creams or lotions (best when only a small area of skin is affected), or as capsules or tablets.

➤ Retin A, derived from vitamin A, can reduce sebum production, and so prevent blackheads and spots. Side-effects, such as redness, irritation and scaling, are quite common. Use the cream sparingly – if excess redness occurs, stop treatment for a few days.

➤ Contraceptives with a high progesterone content may aggravate acne, including some types of the combined pill. Switching to an alternate preparation may help, particularly the combined pill Dianette. This contains an anti-androgen hormone, cyproterone acetate. It's particularly useful for women with acne associated with polycystic ovarian syndrome (see page 144).

➤ Roaccutane is a more powerful vitamin A derivative that can really help even severe cases of acne. However, side-effects are common, and potentially serious. It can also damage a growing foetus, so pregnancy must be avoided during treatment, and for three months afterwards. Because it can be so dangerous, Roaccutane can only be prescribed by hospital specialists.

ACQUIRED IMMUNE DEFICIENCY SYNDROME (AIDS)

This devastating illness, which slowly destroys the immune system of the body, is caused by human immuno-deficiency viruses (or HIV). It used to be regarded as an illness mainly of homosexual men, but this is no longer the case. Worldwide, more women are affected than men, and in this country increasing numbers of women are being infected, predominantly through either sexual intercourse, or from drug abuse using contaminated needles. Having sex with a bisexual man is likely to pose the greatest risk, but many women have been infected via sex with heterosexual men. The virus is present in the semen of infected men, and during intercourse it has an easy route into a woman's body through the womb lining. During pregnancy, the virus can pass into, and infect, the baby. Breast feeding after birth increases this risk. Symptoms of the infection appear anything between one and ten years after the initial infection. On average, the time between the initial infection and the development of serious complications is eight to ten years. Though modern drugs can help to boost the immune system, improve quality of life and prolong survival, once AIDS is established, it is eventually virtually always fatal. There are a few very rare cases of HIV infected children later becoming HIV negative, but so far this has never been known to occur in adults.

The first symptoms of HIV infection include:
➤ swollen lymph nodes
➤ skin rashes, including greasy, flaky skin on the face, ringworm and multiple boils
➤ herpes and shingles
➤ recurrent bouts of diarrhoea and weight loss.

The initial phase of the illness, known as Aids Related Complex (or ARC) can last many months or years. Eventually it progresses to AIDS, with the occurrence of a serious, life-threatening infection, or cancer, as the immune system becomes increasing damaged. This damage can be measured in the form of the numbers of a certain type of white cell, known as CD4, present in the blood stream. A CD4 count of less than 200 is suggestive of full-blown AIDS.

In AIDS, unusual infections occur which the body is unable to fight. These include:
➤ pneumonia caused by variety of organisms, including TB and pneumocytis
➤ infection by the Cytomegalovirus, or CMV, causing pneumonia, brain inflammation, eye damage and severe sweating
➤ widespread fungal infections on the skin, in the mouth and bowel

➤ severe herpes
➤ an unusual type of skin cancer, known as Kaposi's sarcoma.
 Treatment for anyone infected with HIV is now offered by doctors working in specialist centres where qualified staff can provide a safe environment and counselling, if required.

The HIV Test
After the HIV virus enters the bloodstream, antibodies are produced against it, though this process may take up to three months. It is these antibodies (and not the virus itself) that are detected in an HIV test. This means that a negative test does not rule out a new infection that could have occurred in the previous three months. A negative test does not mean that you are immune to HIV. You could still become infected if you put yourself at risk. A positive result, on the other hand, does not mean that you have AIDS. However, it does mean that you are infectious, and can pass the virus to other people through unprotected sex. But you can't infect someone by hugging, kissing, drinking, eating, working or sharing a house with other people.

Preventing the transmission of HIV
At the moment there is no vaccine against HIV, but the spread of the disease can be prevented by some simple precautions:
➤ Practise safer sex. This means using condoms every time you have sex, especially if you have a new partner. This applies even if you are on the Pill. If he's not prepared to use a condom, then don't have sex with him! Female condoms (Femidom) are probably as effective as ordinary men's condoms, but this has not been proved as yet
➤ If you use a lubricant, make sure it is water-based, such as K-Y jelly. Oil-based lubricants, such as Vaseline or baby oil, can damage the rubber in condoms, rendering them unsafe for contraception as well as preventing infections
➤ Using a spermicide can help give further protection, as it kills off HIV as well as sperm (but using spermicide on its own is not particularly effective)
➤ Anal sex is more risky than vaginal sex, as the friction can cause abrasions in the anal canal, which is an easy route for the virus to enter the body
➤ Open sores, such as a cut or herpes on the vulva, increase the risk of the virus entering your body
➤ The more sexual partners you have, the greater the risk. Having unprotected sex just once with an infected man could prove a fatal mistake.

AGEING

Increasing age brings both physical and mental changes to the body. Though ageing is a gradual process, in women the changes tend to be more noticeable in the fifth decade, after the menopause (see page 120). The skin becomes less elastic and more wrinkled (especially if it has been exposed to a lot of sunlight, see page 157), and the muscles become weaker. Bones become thinner (osteoporosis, see page 128) and joints can become worn, with stiffness and pain (osteoarthritis, see page 17).

Circulation can become sluggish and the heart less efficient, leading to more noticeable shortness of breath during exercise (heart disease, page 93). There is also a gradual loss of cells in the nervous system, leading to a reduced memory in some people. All these changes are accelerated by smoking, prolonged excessive use of alcohol, a lack of physical exercise and a poor diet.

ALCOHOL

It's easy to forget that alcohol is a very powerful drug. Even small amounts (one or two units) can cause a change in the functioning of the brain, and chronic long-term abuse can cause permanent damage to the liver, heart and nervous system. It can also be a factor in causing high blood pressure, and increases the risk of cancers of the liver, mouth, throat and oesophagus (the food pipe). Drinking even moderate amounts of alcohol (three or more units regularly each day) during pregnancy can also cause severe, permanent damage to the growing baby.

However, there's now evidence that drinking small amounts of alcohol can actually be good for your health. In particular, it can reduce the risk of developing heart disease. Women who are at high risk of heart disease from other causes, such as smoking, or obesity, are likely to benefit most from regular light drinking, particularly wine (one or two units per day). However, women are far more susceptible than men to the harmful effects of alcohol, and it's important not to drink more than twenty units per week – some doctors say that fourteen is quite enough.

However, every woman who drinks regularly should be aware that alcohol can be very addictive, and it's very easy to become dependent on it, gradually drinking larger amounts each day.

Warning signs for a possible drinking problem include:
➤ thinking you need to cut down on your drinking
➤ having someone criticise you for drinking too much

A

ALCOHOLIC DRINKS – UNITS OF ALCOHOL

Beer, lager and cider		Fortified wine	
Half pint (284ml, 10fl oz)		1 pub measure	
Bitter	1	(50ml, $^1/_3$ gill)	
Brown ale	1	Dry sherry or similar	1
Strong ale or lager	2	Medium sherry	1
Low-alcohol lager	0.25	Cream sherry	1
Dry cider	1		
Sweet cider	1	**Spirits**	
Strong cider	2	1 single measure	
		(25ml, $^1/_6$ gill*)	
Wine		Brandy, whisky, gin,	
Average small glass		rum or vodka	1
(113ml, 4fl oz)			
Dry white wine	1	* Northern Ireland and some parts	
Rosé	1	of Scotland serve larger measures	
Sweet white wine	1	($^1/_4$ gill) which counts as $1^1/_2$	
Champagne	1	units each	

➤ feeling guilty about your drinking
➤ needing an 'eye-opener' first thing in the morning

You definitely have a problem if:
➤ you always need to have alcohol to hand, and get anxious when there's none available
➤ you have got into trouble, or have had job or marital problems, because of your drinking
➤ you keep having to increase the amount you drink to feel the effect
➤ until you've had your first drink of the day you feel sick, irritable or sweaty, or have the shakes.

Self-help
If you are only drinking a little bit too much, then you may be able to get your drinking under control by simply deciding to cut down and sticking to it. Tell your friends and relatives what you are doing, so that they don't encourage you to drink more than you want to. Try and identify when you are most likely to drink – for instance, when you go to the pub with friends, or when you're feeling lonely in the evenings – then take positive steps to avoid alcohol at these times.

But don't be afraid to seek professional help if you can't break the habit on your own.

Help from professionals
Your GP can help by either offering support and counselling in the surgery, or referring you to a specialist centre. This could be either a unit attached to an NHS hospital, or an independent counselling and advice centre. If you prefer, you can also go to many of these without a referral letter. They are usually listed in the local telephone directory, under 'alcohol'. Their advice should be free.

Prevention
Alcohol dependence can often be prevented by:
➤ drinking slowly, and not gulping. Don't drink alcohol if you're thirsty, have a soft drink first instead
➤ don't drink on an empty stomach
➤ don't drink to relieve anxiety, tension and depression
➤ never feeling embarrassed about refusing an alcoholic drink.

ALLERGIES
An allergy is caused by an over reaction of the body's own immune system to a substance that is usually harmless. Allergies commonly affect the skin, causing eczema and dermatitis; the nose and airway, causing hayfever, rhinitis, and asthma; and the stomach and intestines, causing digestive problems. Sometimes, contact with an offending substance can trigger a severe reation throughout the body, leading to a swelling of the skin and lining of the airway, and shock, which very occasionally can be fatal.

The most common substances that cause allergic reactions in the airway are pollen grains, the house dust mite, animal fur and excretions. Common foods causing digestive allergic reactions are dairy products, eggs, fish (especially shellfish) and red fruits (especially strawberries). Perfume – either on its own, or in cosmetics, skin creams and bath additives – is a common cause of allergic skin rashes in women.

Many people inherit a tendency to allergic reactions, a condition known as atopy.

Self-help for allergic reactions
➤ Avoid contact with known trigger substances as much as possible.

➤ Anti-histamine tablets, eye drops and nasal sprays can ease hayfever symptoms.
➤ Skin rashes can be eased by applying 1 percent hydrocortisone cream. In severe cases, taking an anti-histamine tablet can also be helpful.
➤ People who have suffered a severe reaction with swelling of the airway, should carry an adrenalin with them at all times, either in the form of an inhaler or an injection.

Help from your docter
➤ Stronger drugs, especially steroids, are available for more severe reactions.
➤ Patch testing can help to identify the cause of severe, repeated allergic reactions. A small amount of several different substances are allied to the skin. Inflammation, with swelling, redness and itching, indicate an allergic reaction.

ANOREXIA NERVOSA

This is a serious eating disorder that's becoming increasingly common. Though it affects mainly teenage girls and young women, more and more cases in men and older women are being reported.

Anorexia nearly always starts as a weight-reducing diet that goes out of control. Instead of returning to normal eating upon reaching a target weight, sufferers have a distorted image of their own body, and see themselves as fat even when they look painfully thin to others. They carry on denying themselves food, and exercise excessively in order to lose more weight. Even when they admit they don't need to lose any more, anorexics have a pathological fear of gaining weight, and so continue on a diet that verges on starvation. It's a genuine and severe mental illness that can be very difficult to treat.

Apart from obvious weight loss, other symptoms include:
➤ no periods. The ovaries 'switch off' once body weight falls below the minimum fat-to-muscle ratio required by the body to produce oestrogen. This in turn can lead to low oestrogen levels, and osteoporosis
➤ dry skin and fine baby-like 'lanugo' hair growing over the body
➤ tiredness and weakness
➤ chronic constipation, which can lead to laxative abuse in severe cases, liver and kidney failure.
Anorexia needs prompt and careful specialist treatment. If you suspect someone has it, then try and persuade them to see a doctor

as soon as possible. However, this can be difficult as many anorexics deny they have a problem, or are scared to seek help, fearing they will be force-fed to make them put on weight. It can be helpful to everyone if you have a chat with the doctor first.

Treatment usually involves intensive psychotherapy, often together with anti-depressants.

In-patient treatment in hospital is used as a last resort. Even after an initial recovery, many anorexics suffer relapses in times of stress, and sadly, up to 10 percent of long-term sufferers die as a result of their illness, either through suicide or starvation.

ANXIETY

It's normal to feel anxious at times – for example, when a relative is ill, when you're about to do an important exam or waiting for the result, or when you are faced with large bills that you can't pay.

But some people feel anxious nearly all of the time, for no good reason. This doesn't just affect emotions – it can cause a wide variety of other symptoms including:
➤ palpitations and chest pains
➤ a tight chest, and a feeling that you can't breathe properly
➤ breathing too fast (hyperventilating), which can cause dizziness and fainting
➤ a constant lump in the throat
➤ nausea and diarrhoea
➤ sweating
➤ a frequent need to pass urine
➤ constant tiredness due to sleepless nights.
Anxiety may occur on its own, or be a part of another mental disorder, such as depression or hypochondria. It's a problem that's twice as common in women than men. Sufferers are often labelled 'neurotic', but anxiety can be so severe that it completely disrupts normal everyday living.

Self-help
Just recognising you have a problem is a great step forward. Simple steps that can really reduce anxiety levels include:
➤ taking regular exercise. This can be a surprisingly good relaxant for the mind and body, and one of the best natural ways of getting a good night's sleep
➤ slowing down. When you're feeling anxious it's easy to get into a panic about getting tasks done, which only makes anxiety worse

Taking tasks at a more leisurely pace will help to calm your mind
➤ make time to relax and do something you enjoy
➤ try and put worrying events in the past to the back of your mind
  Learn to live in the present, not in the past
➤ avoid drinking too much coffee, tea, or cola. The caffeine they
  contain can make anxiety worse. Avoid excessive amounts of
  alcohol too. Though small amounts can be a relaxant, in large
  amounts it can cause depression, and make anxiety worse
➤ some essential aromatherapy oils can help to relieve anxiety,
  such as lavender, geranium and sandalwood. They are particularly effective when used for massage (which in itself can help
  relieve anxiety) or alternatively, as a bath additive.

Help from your doctor
Don't be scared or ashamed to seek help if anxiety is threatening to
take over your life.

The best treatment for anxiety is counselling or psychotherapy. A
professional counsellor can help to both identify any underlying
reasons for the problem, and also give practical training in dealing
with it effectively, including relaxation techniques.

Drugs that can be used for anxiety include:
➤ beta-blockers, which can help to stop many of the unpleasant
  physical symptoms, such as sweating, tremors, and palpitations.
  Beta-blockers should not be taken by people with asthma .
➤ tranquillizers, such as diazepam. These are very effective at
  reducing anxiety, but are very addictive. They should only
  be used for a real crisis, and then for a maximum of five days at
  a time
➤ some anti-depressants can be effective, particularly where
  anxiety is part of a depressive illness. Unlike tranquillizers, they
  aren't addictive.

ARTHRITIS
Arthritis causes painful, stiff and swollen joints.There are two main
types – osteoarthritis, caused by 'wear and tear', and inflammatory
arthritis, caused by damage from the body's own immune system.
Both are more common in women than men.

OSTEOARTHRITIS
This is the most common form of arthritis, especially in older women
and is due to the joint surfaces simply becoming rough and worn.

Weight-bearing joints, such as the hips and knees, are often the worst affected. It can also affect the joints between the bones that make up the spine, especially in the neck and the lower back (see page 21 on back pain).

However, any joint that does a lot of work can be affected by osteoarthritis. In women who do a lot of housework or typing, it's often the finger joints that show the first signs of wear.

The first symptom of osteoarthritis is usually aching, especially first thing in the morning. In many cases, the disease never progresses beyond this. But if a joint does become more worn it becomes more painful, and may also become swollen. Finger joints can become noticeably knobbly, making it difficult to get rings on and off.

Though some wear and tear is inevitable with increasing age, osteoarthritis is more likely if you are overweight, as this puts a greater strain on the joints. Thin, osteoporotic bones are also more susceptible to damage.

Self-help
➤ Ease the strain on your joints by keeping your weight down.
➤ Take gentle exercise to prevent stiffness, but avoid heavy, weight-bearing exercise, such as running, which can make the problem worse. Swimming is best, as the water provides support.
➤ Eat plenty of calcium to keep your bones strong, and consider hormone-replacement therapy (HRT) after the menopause.
➤ Keep yourself warm in winter. Wear thick gloves and tights when you go outside. Cold always makes joint pain and stiffness worse.
➤ Simple paracetamol can ease mild pain, but for more severe pain try a painkiller containing codeine as well. Anti-inflammatory painkillers, such as Ibuprofen, can ease stiffness too, and can be taken in addition to paracetamol.
➤ A daily supplement of cod liver oil can help to lubricate stiff joints (and help to prevent heart disease!).

Help from your doctor
➤ Stronger painkillers are available on prescription.
➤ Physiotherapy can be really helpful for stiff, aching joints.
Sadly, there's no cure for a worn joint, other than replacement by an artificial one. However, artificial joints have a limited lifespan, and the operation can have risks, so it's generally reserved for severe, disabling osteoarthritis.

INFLAMMATORY ARTHRITIS

This includes rheumatoid arthritis (the most common), and arthritis linked to disease caused by a defective immune system, such as Crohn's disease.

Crohn's disease is a type of arthritis that can affect people of all ages, including children and teenagers. The body's own immune system attacks the lining of joints, causing severe inflammation and eventually permanent structural damage.

Rheumatoid arthritis can affect any joint in the body, especially the shoulders, wrists, fingers, knees and neck joints. They become stiff and painful, look swollen, and feel warm to touch. Rheumatoid arthritis can also cause general tiredness and malaise.

Diagnosis is by blood tests, which your GP can arrange. In mild cases, self-treatment with anti-inflammatory painkillers may be sufficient to control pain and stiffness. However, because rheumatoid arthritis can be a progressive disease, flare-ups of inflammation are best treated by a doctor. More severe disease is treated by regular physiotherapy (to ease stiffness) together with powerful immuno-suppressant drugs, including steroids.

ASTHMA

At least three million people in the UK suffer from asthma. Though the illness is more common in children, at least one in twenty women are affected. It's caused by inflammation and subsequent narrowing in the airways in the lungs, leading to wheezing and shortness of breath.

Often there is no obvious cause for asthma attacks, but in many cases, attacks are triggered by:
➤ smoking, and other environmental pollutants
➤ colds, and other respiratory infections
➤ exercise
➤ cold air
➤ some drugs
➤ anxiety and stress.

Symptoms can vary between slight wheezing, with a dry cough, especially at night, to severe shortness of breath, with severe wheezing, and difficulty in breathing.

Prevention

Unfortunately, there is no known cure yet for asthma, but many attacks can be prevented:

➤ Stop smoking. Asthmatics should also try and avoid going into smoky or polluted areas. This includes city centres full of traffic fumes, especially on hot summer days, when high pollen counts can add to the problem
➤ Many asthma attacks are triggered by the house dust mite, which thrives in feather pillows and mattresses. Always use synthetic bed linen, and cover mattresses with a synthetic protector. All upholstery and curtains should be vacuumed regularly to keep general dust levels as low as possible
➤ Keep stress levels down by learning to relax and taking regular exercise – yes, this is possible, even for asthmatics!
➤ Use 'preventer' drugs regularly
➤ People who tend to have severe attacks, especially associated with infections, should have a flu vaccination each year in the autumn.

Treatment
Most drugs used to treat asthma are given in the form of a powder, which is inhaled into the lungs. Small pressurized cans, or inhalers, are the most common type of device used, but powder can also be inhaled from special capsules, or from a disc.

For more severe cases where a patient cannot use an inhaler device, drugs can be given by mouth, or in emergencies, in inhaled droplet form, via a nebulizer machine.

There are two main types of treatment for asthma
➤ 'Reliever' drugs help to widen narrowed airways. They should be used occasionally during an asthma attack, but only severe asthmatics should need to use them on a regular basis. The most common one used in salbutamol. Most asthma attacks can be prevented before they ever start by using
➤ 'Preventer' drugs, which help to stop the airways narrowing. They should be used regularly each day, even if there is no wheezing. The most common are inhaled steroids.
All asthmatics should have a check-up with their doctor at least once a year, or if attacks occur frequently, once a month.

B

BACKACHE

At some time four out of five women can expect to suffer from back pain that's bad enough to necessitate sick leave from work. The good news is that no matter what the cause, in 90 percent of cases, back pain gets better of its own accord, usually within a few days.

The backbone is made up of twenty-four separate bones, called vertebrae, held together by strong ligaments and muscles. In between the vertebrae are fibrous discs, each with a soft, spongy centre. The backbone acts as a main support for the body, and also protects the spinal cord. This important structure carries nerve impulses from the brain and transmits them to the rest of the body, via the spinal nerves, which leave the cord in between each pair of vertebrae.

Muscular strain is by far the most common cause of back pain, especially in younger women. It's caused by extra stress on the spine, either through lifting heavy objects, bad posture, pregnancy, or from being overweight. The pain is usually a deep ache in the lower back, which can spread to involve the buttocks and thighs as well.

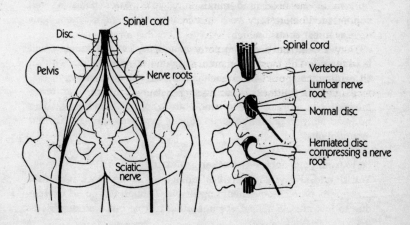

A slipped disc causes severe pain in the back The disk, placing pressure on a nearby spinal nerve can cause a shooting pain down into the buttock and outer thigh, which may spread down as far as the outside edge of the foot. It is not actually the disc that slips, but the lining that ruptures, causing the jelly-like substance inside the disc to escape, and press on the spinal nerves. Disc problems tend to occur mainly in younger people as a result of a violent movement in sports, or from very heavy lifting. In older people it occurs because of general wear causing weakness in the disc structure.

In older women, back pain is often caused by osteo-arthritis, whereby the joints between the vertebrae become inflamed and worn. Osteoporosis only causes backache in the advanced stages, when the bones are so fragile that they collapse. Lower backache can also be caused by a kidney infection and gynaecological problems. Much more rarely, it can be due to secondary deposits from cancer, particularly breast cancer.

Self-help
The traditional treatment for all types of back pain has always been to rest horizontally on a firm surface – either the floor or a very firm bed – for several days until the pain eases. Though this may be appropriate for disc problems, there is increasing evidence that muscular tension is more likely to ease with continued gentle movement and activity. However, anyone with lower backache should avoid sitting down as much as possible, as this puts an extra strain on the lower-back muscles. If you can't avoid sitting, then sit as upright as possible, and make sure your lower back is well supported, if necessary with a rolled-up towel or cushion. This applies to car seats too.

Simple analgesics, such as paracetamol, aspirin and codeine, will take the edge off most back pain, but generally painkillers with an anti-inflammatory action, such as ibuprofen, are more effective.

A hot bath followed by a massage, can help to loosen up tense muscles. Use either a moisturising body lotion, or even better, some body oil with an additional few drops of lavender and sandalwood essential oils.

Help from your doctor and other professionals
You should always seek medical advice for severe back pain that makes any type of movement impossible. Though this could well be due to just muscle spasm, it's important to rule out a more serious

cause. Strong prescription-only painkillers and muscle relaxants can ease the pain.

You should also see a doctor straight away if you have back pain and lose control of your bladder or bowels.

Physiotherapy, osteopathy, chiropractic and acupuncture are usually more effective for treating back pain than taking tablets. If you decide to self-refer yourself privately to avoid a long wait, make sure the practitioner is fully qualified.

X-rays and more detailed magnetic resonance imaging (MRI) scans can help to determine the cause of persistent bouts of severe pain. MRI scans produce a high-quality image using magnetism and radio waves instead of X-rays.

Many disc problems do get better on their own, but for severe cases, surgery can be performed to relieve pressure on the spinal nerves.

Prevention

Most back problems can be prevented by:

➤ always bending at the knees when you do any lifting – this includes babies and toddlers as well as household equipment and bags of shopping
➤ sleeping on a firm bed that supports the curve of your spine
➤ taking regular general exercise to keep fit, and doing regular back exercises to keep your muscles supple
➤ if you work at a desk, check that the chair (and any typing or computer equipment) is at the right height and position
➤ use a trolley for heavy loads whenever you can.

BARTHOLIN'S GLANDS

These are two small glands at the entrance to the vagina. During sexual arousal they secrete a clear fluid, which aids lubrication during intercourse.

Occasionally the duct from one of the glands becomes blocked, leading to the formation of a Bartholin's cyst. These often drain spontaneously, but have a habit of recurring, in which case surgery is required to cure the problem. If one of these cysts becomes infected, an acutely painful abscess can form. This is best treated by immediate surgery to drain the pus.

B

BLADDER PROBLEMS
See Cystitis (page 46) and Incontinence (page 103).

BLOATING
A bloated abdomen can be caused by:
➤ excess gas in the bowels
➤ indigestion, often linked with excess stomach acid
➤ constipation
➤ irritable bowel syndrome (page 116)
➤ excessive amounts of dietary fibre
➤ fluid retention, especially before a period
➤ weight gain – fat collects inside your abdomen as well as on the outside
➤ occasionally food intolerance and allergy
➤ occasionally, more serious digestive problems, such as gallstones, or diverticulitis.

Self-help
➤ Try and identify the cause in your case. Keep a diet diary to check for foods that trigger your symptoms.
➤ Eat slowly with your mouth shut. Avoid carbonated drinks.
➤ Eat enough fibre to keep your bowels regular, but no more than this. Cut down on pulses and vegetables that cause gas, such as broccoli and cauliflower.
➤ Tackle pre-menstrual fluid retention by cutting down on salty foods and all caffeine-laden drinks, such as cola and coffee.
➤ Tackle any weight problem by going on a sensible diet.
➤ Take regular exercise – a little every day if possible.
If these don't help, see your doctor. Very occasionally a bloated abdomen can be a sign of a more serious illness, such as an enlarged womb, or an ovarian cyst.

BLOOD PRESSURE
The pressure exerted by the flow of blood through the main arteries is recorded as two measurements. The higher level, the systolic pressure, is the force of the blood as it's pumped out of the heart. The lower measurement, or diastolic pressure, is the pressure in the arteries as the heart relaxes or fills, and signifies the 'resting' pressure inside the main arteries.

A healthy young adult will have a blood pressure of approximately

110/70, but anything between 100/60 and 130/85 is quite normal. Values under 90/50 are usually considered low, and above 140/90 high for people under 60. However, blood pressure does increase naturally with age and 160/100 is normal for a person over 70.

Low blood pressure is a rare condition. It usually causes no symptoms at all, but it can cause a tendency to easy fainting, especially in hot weather, or during pregnancy. It's often considered a sign of good health, and treatment with drugs is not usually given in this country (drugs are used more often in France and Germany to treat low blood pressure). It tends to correct itself with increasing age. Symptoms can often be eased by drinking plenty of fluids during the summer, or before and after vigorous exercise.

High blood pressure (or hypertension) is much more common, especially among older people. It affects between 10 and 20 percent of women, though many are completely unaware they have it! Hypertension tends not to cause any obvious symptoms, although at very high levels it can cause headaches, giddiness, chest pains and blurred vision. It is however a serious health condition. It puts an added strain on the heart, which can lead to heart failure; it increases the risk of having a stroke; and it can damage the arteries, particularly those supplying the kidneys (leading to kidney failure) and those in the eye, leading to sight problems. The higher the pressure, the greater the risks. In many cases, there's no obvious cause for high blood pressure, although it can sometimes be avoided by a general healthy lifestyle, and following the self-help steps below. Sometimes drugs, such as the combined contraceptive pill, are to blame. High blood pressure can also occur during pregnancy, but in most cases it gradually returns to normal after the baby is born.

Self-help for high blood pressure
By adjusting your lifestyle it's often possible to lower your own blood pressure.
➤ High blood pressure can be caused by excess weight. Go on a sensible diet and make a real effort to get down to a medically healthy weight.
➤ Smoking can aggravate high blood pressure. Yet another reason to stop!
➤ Excess alcohol can also increase blood pressure. All women should drink no more than fourteen units a week (see page 13).
➤ Cut down on salt intake as much as possible – there is evidence

that excess salt can raise blood pressure. Don't add salt to your food and avoid salty foods such as salted nuts, crisps, and smoked meats. Many processed foods also contain a large amount of salt.

➤ Take regular exercise. Just half an hour of moderate exercise each day could make a significant difference to both your blood pressure and your general sense of well-being.

➤ Take positive steps to reduce your stress levels. Make sure you have some relaxation time each day.

Monitors for measuring your own blood pressure can be bought from chemists. These can be helpful – especially if you get anxious and your blood pressure shoots up every time you go to see your doctor! But don't let the machine rule your life – there's rarely any need to measure your own blood pressure more than once a week.

Help from your doctor
All people with high blood pressure (even if it's only borderline) should have regular check-ups with either their doctor, or the practice nurse. Hypertension can sometimes be controlled by self-help measures alone, but your doctor is the best person to judge when drug treatment is indicated.

A large range of drugs are available that can help to reduce blood pressure, such as diuretics, beta-blockers, and others known as ACE inhibitors and calcium antagonists! Sometimes a combination of drugs is required to get blood pressure adequately controlled. Unfortunately, many of the drugs can have unwanted side-effects and you may need to try several different drugs before you find one that suits you. As always, don't chop and change too quickly – give each one at least a three-month trial.

High blood pressure usually requires long-term (and sometimes lifelong!) treatment. Never stop your drugs unless your doctor says it's safe to do so!

BREASTS
Each of your breasts consist of glandular tissue and fat. The milk-producing glands drain into one of the fifteen to twenty ducts, which open out on the nipple. Most women have a remarkably similar amount of glandular tissue in their breasts – it's the fat content that is more important in determining your breast size.

The fat and glandular tissue are supported by strong bands of fibrous tissue that pass from the underlying chest muscles, through to the breast skin. Unfortunately, once these bands are stretched, no amount of exercise can shrink them back again, which is why a large increase in your breast size, for instance during pregnancy, breast feeding, or weight gain, can lead to a permanent change in your breast shape. Exercise, however, can help to build up the underlying pectoral muscles.

Breasts are normally the first part of the body to show signs of puberty, and they start to develop at around age eleven. One breast may grow faster than the other and, though big differences are usually evened out by the time full sexual maturity is reached aged sixteen to eighteen, many women will always have one breast that's slightly bigger than the other, and this is quite normal.

Breasts change at different times in our lives. Changing hormone levels in the week before each period leads to fluid retention, making the breast tissue slightly more lumpy and tender. Wearing a supportive bra, night and day, can be helpful. The hormones in the combined contraceptive pill can also cause a slight increase in breast size, and in some cases tenderness as well. If this is very noticeable, changing formulation often helps.

During sex, it's normal for the nipples to become more erect, and for a red flush to appear over the front of the chest and over the breasts. At the menopause, the monthly breast changes stop, and there may be some shrinkage of the breast tissue. These changes are less noticeable in women who take hormone-replacement therapy (HRT).

Pregnancy and breast-feeding
During pregnancy, there's often a very noticeable increase in breast size and tenderness within the first three months. The skin around the nipple (the areola), darkens permanently, and as pregnancy progresses, the veins on the surface of each breast become much more visible. Milk may leak from the nipples during the last three months, although this varies between different women.

After birth, a sudden increase in the hormone, prolactin, stimu-lates milk production, which is then maintained by regular suckling on the nipple. The breasts often feel painfully sore and full for a few days in the first week, until a feeding pattern is established. If you don't breast-feed, the milk will gradually be reabsorbed. Though the drug, bromocriptine, will stop breast-milk production, it's only prescribed to treat severely engorged breasts.

B

TAKING CARE OF YOUR BREASTS
Choosing the right bra

A correctly fitting bra is vital not only for your own comfort, but also for providing the best possible support for your breasts. Large department stores will usually have someone available to measure you for a bra – it's reckoned that more than half of all British women are wearing the wrong size.

There are two parts of a bra size:

❶ measure around your rib cage just underneath your breasts. Add on four inches. This is your basic bra size, such as 34, 36, 38 etc. If it works out at an odd number, for example 35, the size smaller (34) may do if there is a large hook adjustment at the back. Otherwise, go to the next size up (36 in this case).

❷ Measure over the fullest part of your breasts. Don't squash them! You may need an extra pair of hands, so get a friend to help.

Now work out the difference between this measurement and your basic size, and this gives your cup size (n.b. measurements are all in inches):

0	– A cup		3 – 3.5	– D cup
1 – 1.5	– B cup		4 – 4.5	– DD cup
2 – 2.5	– C cup		5 – 5.5	– E cup

Breast self-examination

Every woman should be breast aware. By examining your own breasts regularly you'll soon get to know what they feel like normally, and that way you'll be able to detect any changes that may need further investigations.

The best time for breast self-examination is just after a period. If you don't have periods, choose a convenient time that you're likely to remember, such as the beginning of each calender month. Don't rush – make sure you have some time alone to do it properly. Many women find that during, or after bathing or showering is a good time.

Here's how to do it:

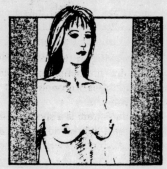

❶ First of all, check the shape of your breasts in a mirror. Has the position of the nipple changed? Does one breast look different from the other?

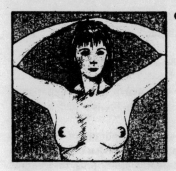

❷ Next, examine the skin of each breast for dimpling, or a change in texture. Do this with your arms by your sides, then with them on your waist, then finally raised above your head, when you should look at the skin of your armpits too.

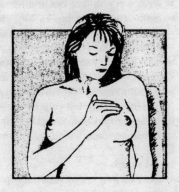

❸ Check the skin of your nipples, then gently squeeze them to check for any unusual discharge.

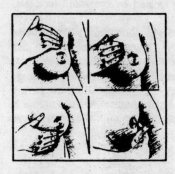

❹ Next, check for lumps. It's best to do this lying down, especially if you have large breasts. Don't squeeze your breasts between the tips of your fingers – press in gently using the flat of your fingers instead. Start at the nipple, and work outwards in circles, extending right up into the armpit on each side.

Remember, if you do find something unusual, don't panic. Most breast lumps are completely benign, and not cancerous, but don't sit around for ages worrying about it. Arrange to see your doctor as soon as you can.

A mammogram is a special X-ray of the breast tissue. It's used to detect breast lumps and to give an indication of whether a lump is cancerous or not. All women aged over fifty should have a mammogram once every three years. An invitation should be sent routinely up until the age of sixty-four – after this you need to ask your doctor to arrange for your screening to continue.

BREAST PROBLEMS
Pain and tenderness
Fluctuating hormone levels mean that many women experience pain and tenderness in either one or both breasts just before a period. To ease this discomfort:
➤ wear a supportive bra at all times, including at night
➤ make sure your bra is big enough, and doesn't squash your breasts. If necessary, have differently sized bras to wear at different times of the month
➤ take a daily supplement of 300mg gammolinolenic acid (GLA) – found in evening primrose oil and starflower oil
➤ if you're on the combined contraceptive pill a change of formulation may help. See your doctor, or family planning nurse.
Your doctor can also prescribe other medications, such as Danazol and Bromocritine, which many women find helpful.

Breast lumps
At least 75 percent of breast lumps are benign (i.e. non-cancerous). Lumps in breast tissue can also be caused by cysts and localized areas of inflammation (mastitis).

The most common type of tumour is a fibroadenoma, which is made up of both glandular and fibrous tissue. They usually feel smooth and mobile, which is why they are often known as a 'breast mouse'.

However, it's impossible for even experienced doctors to diagnose the nature of a breast lump by feel alone. All breast lumps should be thoroughly investigated, which usually involves taking a tiny biopsy, under local anaesthetic, using a fine needle. If a lump is found to be a cyst, the fluid can be drained in a similar way.

BREAST CANCER
The statistics about breast cancer in this country are horrifying.

Each year, nearly 30,000 women in the UK are diagnosed with breast cancer. It's the biggest cause of death in women between the ages of thirty-five and fifty-four.

Breast cancer becomes more common the older you become. It's rare in young women under thirty, but is much more common in the over-60s.

Overall, one in twelve women in this country will suffer from breast cancer at some time in her life. But you are at increased risk if:

➤ one or more of your close relatives has had breast cancer, especially if they suffered before the menopause
➤ you never have children
➤ you have your first baby age thirty or more
➤ your periods start at a young age (ten or less)
➤ you have a late menopause
➤ you are overweight and eat a high fat diet.

There is also some evidence that women who take the combined pill for many years at a young age or who take hormone-replacement therapy (HRT) for more than eight years may be more at risk.

But there's some good news too! Starting your family in your twenties, and breast-feeding your babies, both help to protect against breast cancer.

Breast cancer isn't always fatal. It can be cured, especially if it's diagnosed and treated in the early stages. That's why breast self-examination, and regular mammmograms in older women are so important.

Though a mammogram, or a breast ultrasound can give an indication of whether a lump is cancerous or not, a biopsy is needed for a definite diagnosis.

To be told you have breast cancer is devastating news for any woman. But please, don't despair. Think positive – 85 percent of women treated in the early stages are still alive five years later.

All breast cancer should now be treated in special breast units, by doctors with extensive training in breast disease. Most patients are treated with surgery of some sort, but thankfully in many cases removal of the whole breast – a mastectomy – isn't necessary. Removing the lump alone can be just as effective, and this often only leaves a tiny scar on the breast, with no obvious change in the breast shape.

Depending on the type, and extent of the tumour, further treatment in the form of radiotherapy or chemotherapy may be required. In addition, many women are also treated with Tamoxifen, which blocks the action of oestrogen on the breast, and can help prevent further tumour growth.

NIPPLE PROBLEMS

The nipples, the darker tips of each breast, mark the position of the openings of between fifteen and twenty milk ducts. The area around the nipple (the areola) is pinkish-brown, but darkens permanently with pregnancy.

B

Nipples have a rich nerve supply, which makes them particularly sensitive to touch, or to temperature changes. Nipples are occasionally naturally turned inwards (or inverted) and this can cause difficulties with breast-feeding. Special nipple shields can help to overcome this problem. New inversion of a nipple should never be ignored, as it can be a sign of breast cancer.

Itchy nipples can be caused by a chafing bra seam (switch to a seamless design), and biological washing powders (switch to washing your bras in non-biological washing powders, or just rinse, or soak in water).

Nipples are also a common site for eczema. Though this usually clears with low strength steroid creams, such as 1 percent hydrocortisone, persistent flaking nipples should always be reported to a doctor. It can be a sign of Pagets disease, caused by a tumour inside a milk duct.

Nipple discharge

The commonest time for nipple discharge is during pregnancy, when a clear yellow discharge often appears after the twentieth week (and sometimes earlier). This is a sign that the milk glands are becoming active, and towards the time the baby is due, the discharge may become more milky. However, not all pregnant women have a nipple discharge, and is in no way an indicator of future milk production!

After weaning, it can be several weeks, and sometimes months, before the breasts finally become dry.

Outside pregnancy, any nipple discharge should be reported to a doctor. A milky discharge can be a sign of an excess of the hormone prolactin, caused by a tumour in the pituitary gland. A blood-stained or green discharge can be caused by a polyp or inflammation in a milk duct, but occasionally can be a sign of cancer.

BREAST SURGERY
Mastectomy

The main reason for removal of the whole of a breast is to treat breast cancer. Radical mastectomy, which also involves removal of some of the underlying chest muscles, is rarely performed these days. Mastectomy usually involves removal of the nipple, leaving a straight scar across the chest wall. Sometimes it's possible to have an implant inserted, either immediately or some months later, which gives a better cosmetic result.

A subcutaneous mastectomy involves removing just the glandular tissue beneath the skin, then immediately replacing it with an implant. The nipple is left in place. This procedure has occasionally been performed to prevent breast cancer in women at very high risk.

Removal of the lymph nodes in the armpit at the same time as a mastectomy can interfere with lymph drainage from the arm, leading to swollen fingers. Exercises and special splints can help relieve the discomfort that this can cause.

Breast reduction

Removal of some breast tissue to reduce breast size is most often performed privately for women who feel heavy chested. But it is occasionally performed free on the NHS for women who are very lop-sided, with one breast larger than the other; who have very large breasts that are disproportionate in size to the rest of their body and are causing postural problems, leading to backache; or for women who feel that the sheer size of their breasts causes difficulty with everyday activities, such as sports.

The operation can lead to loss of nipple sensitivity, and can also can make breast-feeding difficult.

Breast augmentation

The desire for a fashionable cleavage has meant that breast enlargement operations using implants are becoming increasingly popular.

Silicone implants give the best cosmetic result, but there are worries that leakage of silicone can cause other illnesses, particularly aching joints and tiredness. The common alternative is saline.

The implant is placed either in front of, or behind, the muscle of the chest. In most cases, there are only three tiny scars afterwards, and most women are able to breast-feed a baby. However, implants can make routine examination of the breast difficult, and may therefore hinder the early detection of breast cancer.

As with all plastic surgery, make sure you are in the hands of a fully qualified surgeon, who has had special plastic surgery training. Your doctor will be able to refer you to a suitable specialist.

BULIMIA

Bulimia is a genuine mental illness which causes bouts of gross over-eating, usually followed by either self-induced vomiting or large quantities of laxatives. The illness often starts in adolescence as a means of weight control, and is far more common in girls than boys. It's thought that at least 10 percent of teenage girls are affected, although in some it's only a sporadic problem that occurs at times of stress. In others, this behaviour pattern becomes increasingly addictive, and can lead to severe health problems. These include eroded teeth, dehydration, kidney failure, fits, and heart disease.

Many bulimia sufferers have also suffered from anorexia at some time as well. However, unlike anorexia, bulimia can often be successfully treated by psychotherapy, together with anti-depressants.

C

CANCER

One in three people will have a cancer diagnosed at some time during their lives, and one in four will eventually die from cancer. Each year, more than 130,000 women are diagnosed as having cancer, and more than 77,000 die from the disease. The most common cancer by far in women is breast cancer (more than 30,000 new cases each year, see page 30), followed by skin (more than 17,000 new cases), then bowel (approximately 15,000 new cases), lung (approximately 13,000 new cases), then ovary and cervix (more than 5,000 cases each).

The earlier cancer is diagnosed, the greater the chance of a cure. All women should become breast aware and examine their own breasts regularly (see page 28). They should also have a smear test, and pelvic examination once very three years.

Prevention

You can help to reduce your risk of cancer by:

➤ not smoking. Smoking is the biggest cancer risk of all, causing 30 percent of all UK cancer deaths. The sooner you stop, the better
➤ eating a healthy diet. This means cutting down on fats, especially animal fats, and eating plenty of fibre, fresh fruit and vegetables. Taking a daily supplement of the anti-oxidant vitamins A, C and E may also be beneficial
➤ avoid drinking too much alcohol
➤ avoiding exposing your skin to strong sunlight. It's especially important to avoid getting burnt
➤ avoiding having unprotected sex with numerous sexual partners.

For information on breast cancer, see page 30, ovarian cancer page 131, cervical cancer, page 40, and, endometrial cancer page 172.

CARPAL TUNNEL SYNDROME

This is a condition causing tingling, pain, weakness and occasionally numbness of the middle fingers of either one or both hands. It's caused by pressure on a nerve as it passes under the tight ligament

C

band at the wrist. It's much more common in women than men, and often occurs for no apparent reason. However, it can be caused by fluid retention, especially during pregnancy, or from premenstrual hormonal changes or occasionally in women starting on the combined pill.

Treatment is with rest and anti-inflammatory drugs. Wearing a supportive elastocrepe bandage is also helpful. A local steroid injection into the wrist may also help to dampen down inflammation. In severe cases, the pressure on the nerve can be relieved by surgically cutting the ligaments around it. Acupuncture and osteopathy may also help.

CELLULITE

This is the term used to describe fat dimply areas of skin, which can resemble orange peel. It's caused by swollen fat cells, and some doctors argue that there is no difference between cellulite and ordinary fat. However, cellulite does have its own unique and troublesome characteristics. The dimpled areas are caused by fibrous bands that run up between the fat cells to the skin surface, and these tend to be more prominent on the buttocks, thighs and occasionally, the upper arms. Cellulite also seems to be remarkably difficult to shift, and although it's more common in women who are generally overweight, it can also affect women of normal weight in localized areas.

Self-help for cellulite
➤ Lose any excess weight by going on a sensible reducing diet. Don't crash diet, as rapid weight loss can cause loose skin, and make dimpling worse. Aim for a steady loss of about 2lb (1kg) each week.
➤ Concentrate on simply cooked, natural foods, with plenty of fresh fruit and vegetables. Especially avoid processed salty foods, such as crisps and meat pies. Apart from being very fattening, they can promote water retention, which makes cellulite worse.
➤ Cut down on tea, coffee and cola. Drink herbal teas and fruit juices instead.
➤ Take regular exercise. This helps to improve the circulation to those stubborn fat cells, and also helps to tone up the underlying muscles. Concentrate on working muscles in the worst affected areas. Though exercise classes or 'working out' with weights in a gym will give results, simple walking or cycling are excellent for thighs, and swimming is good for the upper arms.

C

➤ Massage affected areas vigorously for at least ten minutes each day. This stimulates the circulation and may help to break down fat cells and eliminate excess tissue fluid.
➤ Be wary of anti-cellulite creams. They may make your skin look firmer, but on their own they won't make your cellulite go away.

Help from your doctor
➤ Taking extra oestrogen can make cellulite worse. If you're on the combined oral contraceptive pill, check with your doctor if it's possible to switch to a lower-dose formulation, or alternatively, switch to the progesterone-only pill, or a barrier method. The dose of oestrogen in most forms of hormone-replacement therapy (HRT) is very low, and is unlikely to have an effect on cellulite, but higher-dose formulations may make it more difficult to lose weight.
➤ As a last resort, the fat can be sucked away surgically, by lipo-suction. However, this can be risky, and leave the skin more pitted than before. Like all cosmetic procedures, it should only be done by a fully trained and experienced surgeon. (see page 44).

THE CERVIX
The cervix, or neck of the womb, is a small, rubbery cylinder, that can be felt at the top of the vagina. Passing through the centre is a small passageway leading into the cavity of the womb. This is where blood passes out from the womb during a period, and where sperm enters the womb after intercourse.

Before pregnancy the opening of the cervical canal is quite narrow, but it changes shape, and remains slightly wider after normal childbirth.

The cells lining the cervical canal secrete mucus and appear red and fragile, while those on the vaginal surface are smooth and firm, and more like skin.

Problems
A cervical erosion is a usually harmless condition whereby cells from the canal are found on the vaginal surface as well. Occasionally this can cause a discharge and bleeding after inter-course, a condition that's more common in women taking the combined contraceptive pill. Treatment, usually by cautery, is only required if an erosion is causing bothersome symptoms such as a

C

discharge. Cautery is careful destruction of a small area of tissue with heat.

Inflammation of the cervix is usually due to infection, particularly with chlamydia and gonorrhoea. Unfortunately, infection of the cervix alone often causes no symptoms, but left untreated the infection can spread up to the womb and fallopian tubes, causing pelvic inflammatory disease (PID, see page 134). The cervix can also be infected with viruses, particularly herpes, and the wart virus (also known as the human papilloma virus, or HPV). Cervical warts may be visible to the naked eye as small white growths, but the infection may only be revealed by a smear test.

Cervical polyps are small, fleshy outgrowths from the cells lining the cervical canal. They can cause bleeding between periods, especially after intercourse. They are commonly the size of a small grape, and are completely benign. They can often be simply twisted off, though the base may need cauterising afterwards to prevent bleeding.

Cervical smear tests
Cancer of the cervix is a common and often lethal condition. This is sad, because unlike many cancers, it can easily be prevented.

The cells of the cervix don't suddenly become cancerous. Abnormalities in the cells occur gradually, and the aim of cervical smear tests is to detect these changes, known as dyskaryosis, in the early stages, so that the cervix can be treated before the cancer has a chance to develop.

A tiny scraping of cells are removed from the cervix, using a special wooden spatula, which are then transferred to a microscope

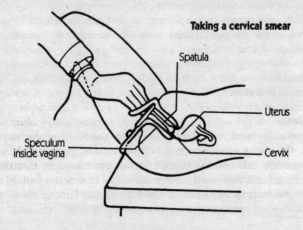

Taking a cervical smear

Spatula

Uterus

Speculum
inside vagina

Cervix

slide and sent to a laboratory for analysis. Occasionally a special sampling brush is used as well.

The test involves lying on a couch whilst the doctor/practice nurse/gynaecologist inserts a metal instrument, called a speculum, into the vagina. Don't be alarmed, it doesn't hurt!

All women should have regular smear tests once they are sexually active (including teenagers). A follow-up test is advisable one year after the first, and if both of these are normal, tests should then be performed at regular three yearly intervals. If any abnormality is detected, more frequent smears may be necessary. All women, up until age sixty-five, should routinely be sent reminders to have a smear by their local health authority, but try to remember yourself when your next test is due – the reminder system doesn't always work as well as it should!

Results

The majority of smear tests are completely normal. However, some women are recalled because there are an inadequate number of cells for analysis on the microscope slide. This is nothing to worry about, and it does not mean there are abnormal cells present. It just means the test needs to be carefully repeated.

Occasionally vaginal infections, such as thrush (see page 164) or trichomonas (see page 169), are also detected on a smear test. Again, although the test may need to be repeated, there is no need to worry. Any abnormal cells, or dyskaryosis, detected on a smear are graded into three main groups. Mild dyskaryosis, as its name suggests, means only slight abnormalities are present. This type of abnormality often reverts back to normal on its own. Treatment is only needed if abnormal cells persist on a follow-up smear six months later.

In moderate and severe dyskaryosis the changes in the cells are more marked, and both need further investigation by colposcopy.

Colposcopy

This is a special magnified examination of the cervix. It involves lying on a couch with special supports to keep the legs wide apart. The gynaecologist exposes the cervix by passing a speculum into the vagina, a metal instrument that holds the walls of the vagina apart. The cervix is then painted with dilute acid, which highlights the abnormal cells, and is viewed by the gynaecologist through a special microscope, placed on a stand at the foot of the bed. Many women find colposcopy a little uncomfortable (and undignified!) but it shouldn't hurt. If it does, say so at once.

C

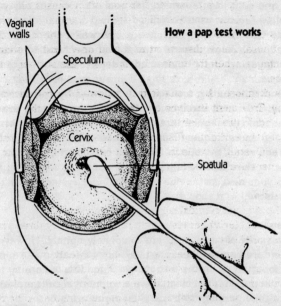

How a pap test works

Vaginal walls

Speculum

Cervix

Spatula

Once the abnormal cells can be seen, a tiny biopsy is taken, to confirm the degree of abnormality. The abnormal cells are then destroyed by either hot diathermy (electric current), freezing (cryosurgery), or by laser. If the abnormal cells extend up into the cervical canal and out of sight of the colposcope, they are removed surgically under anaesthetic by cutting away a cone of tissue – a cone biopsy.

It's essential to have a smear test three to six months after any treatment to confirm that all the abnormal cells have been removed, and frequent smears (at least once a year) for the following five years.

CANCER OF THE CERVIX
More than 5,000 women are still diagnosed each year with cervical cancer. It can occur at any age, and recently there has been an alarming increase in the number of cases in young women under thirty-five.

Cervical cancer is more common in women who have had a genital infection with certain types of wart virus, and women who have had genital warts have a one in three chance of developing abnormal cervical cells. Cervical cancer is also more common in smokers, and in those who have become sexually active at a young age.

C

In the early stages, cervical cancer often causes no symptoms. Later on, it can cause a blood-stained vaginal discharge, and unexpected bleeding, such as in between periods, or after the menopause. Pelvic discomfort and pain only tend to occur in the later stages, when the tumour has spread to the surrounding pelvic organs.

It's diagnosed by a smear test, followed by colposcopy and a biopsy. Treatment involves removal of the womb, the ovaries and surrounding tissues, often followed by chemotherapy. As with all cancers, the earlier the diagnosis is made, the greater the chance of a cure. Overall, more than 50 perent of women treated for cervical cancer survive at least five years.

Prevention
To help prevent cervical cancer all women should
➤ have regular smear tests, preferably once every three years
➤ stop smoking
➤ delay having sex till at least the age of twenty
➤ use barrier contraception, such as a condom or cap
➤ avoid promiscuity. Though some women get cancer after
  only one partner, having several partners increases the risk
  of wart virus infection.

CHLAMYDIA
Chlamydia are small organisms, sized in-between a bacteria and virus. They are a major cause of pelvic inflammatory disease, and subsequent infertility in women.

In men, chlamydia cause non-specific urethritis (NSU), which usually leads to symptoms such as pain on urination, and a discharge from the penis. But in women, genital infection with chlamydia may occasionally cause a vaginal discharge, but often cause no symptoms at all until the infection has spread to, and damaged, the fallopian tubes.

To make matters worse, chlamydial infection cannot be detected by the ordinary vaginal swabs that most GP's use – a special swab is required. In practice, this means that many infections go undetected.

All women with either proven or suspected chlamydial infection, and that means any women who has had sex with a man with NSU, should have prompt treatment. Antibiotics such as tetracyclines or erythromycin (but not penicillin) usually give a rapid cure.

CHLOASMA

This is the name given to pale brown blotches that can occur on the skin of the forhead, cheeks and nose. They are often caused by the hormone oestrogen, and commonly appear during pregnancy. They may also appear in some women taking the combined pill, and are more noticeable if the skin is exposed to the sun. They usually fade once oestrogen levels return to normal.

CHOLESTEROL

This is a fat-like material, known as a lipo-protein, which is an important component of many body cells and is also necessary for the production of some hormones and bile salts (vital for normal digestion).

There are two main types of cholesterol, low-density lipo-protein (LDL) and high-density lipo-protein (HDL). High levels of LDL in the blood stream can lead to fatty deposits (atheroma) forming on the linings of arteries, leading in turn to an increased risk of heart disease and strokes. HDL, on the other hand, seems to have a protective effect.

Nearly all people with a high blood cholesterol level also have a high levels of dangerous LDL. High blood cholesterol is commonly due to simply a poor diet, but some people inherit a tendency to very high levels. Anyone who has had several close family members suffer an early heart attack should always have a cholesterol check. All people should aim to have a cholesterol less than 5.2mmol/l, but those who are at increased risk from heart disease for other reasons (such as smokers, or those with high blood pressure) should aim for an even lower level.

Blood cholesterol levels can usually be controlled by avoiding foods containing a high proportion of saturated fats, such as fatty meats, butter, cheese and eggs, but those with very high levels may need additional drug treatment.

THE CLITORIS

This is the female equivalent of the penis. It's a very small oval-shaped organ just below the pubic bone, at the top of the vulva, above the opening from the bladder. Like the penis, it becomes erect during sexual arousal, and when stimulated in the right way, can lead to an orgasm (see page 128).

CONSTIPATION

This is the infrequent passage of hard, small motions. Anyone can be affected (even children), but it's much more common in women than men, mainly because women eat less bulk and fibre in their daily food.
Symptoms:
➤ straining to pass a motion
➤ passing hard, small stools
➤ passing large amounts of wind (may be very smelly, due to stagnant waste in the bowel)
➤ a bloated uncomfortable tummy
➤ a reduced appetite.

Self-help
Most cases of constipation can be easily cured.
➤ Eat more fibre. The best source is unprocessed bran. It's cheap, and available from most chemists and supermarkets. Start with a couple of dessertspoonfuls sprinkled on a wholewheat cereal each morning, such as weetabix. Or use it with other foods or recipes, such as in cakes, pastry or soups.
➤ Switch to wholemeal bread and pasta, and wholegrain rice. Other good sources of fibre are pulses, such as baked beans, and fresh fruit and vegetables.
➤ Go to the toilet regularly. Don't ignore the urge 'to go'.
➤ Take more exercise, as this can stimulate sluggish bowels.
➤ If these measure don't help, try taking a medicine that naturally bulks up the stools, such as Fybogel or Lactulose. You can buy these directly from chemists.
➤ Avoid stimulant laxatives, such as senna. These purge the bowel, (and that means there's nothing to pass for the next day or so), and if used regularly, can cause a permanently lazy bowel.
➤ Drink more water. This helps to prevent stools becoming dry and compacted.
➤ Abdominal massage in a clockwise direction can help stimulate peristaltic action. Acupressure can help too.
➤ Acupuncture and/or shiatsu treatment can help improve bowel function.
Constipation can be a symptom of Irritable Bowel Syndrome (see page 116), and occasionally a sign of a more serious bowel disorder, such as a polyp or cancer. See your doctor for further advice if your symptoms persist, if you have recurrent bouts of pain or if you have blood in your motions.

CONTRACEPTION

C

(see Family Planning page 68.)

COSMETIC SURGERY

A wide variety of surgical procedures can now be performed to enhance and improve a woman's appearance. The results may either be temporary or permanent.

Though most cosmetic surgery is only performed privately, occasionally certain procedures are performed free on the NHS. These can include:

➤ insertion of breast implants following a mastectomy for breast cancer
➤ corrective surgery to improve the appearance of any part of the body, but particularly the face, after radical surgery for cancer
➤ corrective surgery after severe burns or other trauma.

Occasionally other cosmetic surgery is also performed free when the patient has good cause to be psychologically upset by a part of their body – for instance, where one breast is clearly much larger than the other; when ears stick out very prominently; or for a very large or misshapen nose. However, though in some cases surgery is clearly needed and is arranged without any difficulty at all, there are plenty of women who have been turned down for NHS surgery because either their GP, their surgeon, or both, did not consider the procedure justified.

Many women do request cosmetic surgery for the wrong reasons. It's not an answer to all life's problems. It won't put an unhappy relationship to rights. And though improving your looks may increase your self-confidence, it won't change your basic personality. It should never be done purely to please someone else – it must be something you want to do for yourself. Don't act on impulse, or in a hurry. Though it may be the best thing you ever do, it may be something you live to regret, so give yourself plenty of time to consider it, and if possible, discuss it fully with close friends and relatives.

Like all forms of surgery, cosmetic surgery can be risky. In particular, it can cause obvious scars, or give an end result that looks far more ugly and unsightly than before. These risks are minimized by going to a fully trained, and well-qualified surgeon, who should explain the operation, and its risks, carefully to you. The best route for this is via a referral, or advice from your GP. If you do decide to go it alone, make sure your surgeon is a fellow of the Royal College of Surgeons (FRCS) and is also a member of the British Association of Aesthetic Plastic Surgeons (see Useful Addresses).

C

COUGHS AND COLDS

Nearly everyone has suffered from either a cough or a cold at some time. Most colds are caused by viruses which infect the lining of the nose, leading to inflammation and a discharge. This in turn causes sneezing, and a constant need for a handkerchief! Several hundred different viruses that can cause colds have been identified, which is why it's possible to get one cold after another. Though you may have developed an immunity to one cold virus, another one can soon take hold. Similarly, most coughs are caused by viruses that infect the throat or upper part of the airway leading to the lungs. Viruses are very difficult to treat – taking antibiotics certainly doesn't help. In most cases, however, the body's own immune system works efficiently, and symptoms clear in about a week.

Self-help
➤ Give you own immune system as much help as possible. Get as much rest as you can, with plenty of early nights.
➤ Avoid vigorous exercise. It will tend to make your symptoms worse.
➤ Eat a good diet, with plenty of fresh fruit and vegetables. Extra Vitamin C may help to boost the immune system, so consider taking a daily supplement.
➤ Decongestants can help to relieve a bunged-up, streaming nose. These are available from chemists either in the form of nasal sprays or tablets. Don't use them for more than a few days at a time, however, as they can cause rebound congestion that's worse than before.
➤ An effective old-fashioned remedy is a steam inhalation. Add a few drops of either menthol, eucalyptus oil, or Friars Balsam to a bowlful of steaming water straight from a freshly boiled kettle. Place your head over the bowl, cover with a clean towel, and slowly inhale the vapour.
➤ Echinacea extract is a traditional herbal remedy that can help relieve cold symptoms.
➤ Sore throats and dry tickly coughs can often be eased by a soothing drink of lemon and honey, which are added to a small glass of warm water.

C

➤ Many effective cough medicines are available directly from chemists. Check with the pharmacist for the one that's best for your symptoms. Many contain pholcodeine, which can really help stop repeated bouts of coughing, but it can also cause constipation.

➤ Smoking destroys the natural cleaning and filter system inside the nose and airways, and allows infective viruses and bacteria to settle and flourish. This not only means that smokers are more at risk of infections, but once they occur, they tend to last longer, and are more difficult to treat.

Help from your doctor
Occasionally a second infection, caused by bacteria, can occur in the sinuses or lungs during, or after, a simple cold. Treatment with antibiotics in these cases is often helpful. See your doctor if:

➤ you develop severe facial pain, despite using decongestants

➤ you develop chest pains, or start coughing up coloured phlegm or sputum

➤ you become short of breath or wheezy

➤ you develop a high temperature for more than three days.

Help for others...
Coughs and colds are very common during the autumn and winter months. One tiny droplet from either a cough or sneeze contains millions of viruses that can easily infect other people. If you've got a cold, it's time to be anti-social. Keep it to yourself by avoiding crowded places, especially buses, shops and trains as much as you can. And if you do sneeze, please, turn your head away from others, and put your hand in front of your mouth.

CYSTITIS

This is an inflammation of the lining of the bladder which causes a need to pass urine frequently, often in very small amounts. Passing the urine is acutely painful – it's been likened to passing small pieces of glass. Lower abdominal pain or discomfort is another common symptom.

Though cystitis can occasionally be caused by stones, or more rarely, a bladder tumour, in the vast majority of cases an infection is to blame. Women suffer from cystitis far more than men, because the urethra, the passage from the bladder to the outside is much shorter. This allows bacteria from the anal and vaginal area to spread easily to the bladder.

Having sex often triggers an attack of cystitis for two reasons – it pushes bugs up into the bladder, and the friction from lovemaking can make the delicate tissues around the urethra inflamed and more prone to infection. In older women, the low levels of oestrogen that occur after the menopause can make the bladder lining thin, and again more prone to infection.

Though cystitis is usually only a minor problem, occasionally the infection can spread to the kidneys, causing pyelonephritis. This is far more serious, as occasionally it can cause scarring and permanent kidney damage.

Self-help for cystitis
At the first sign of symptoms:
➤ drink plenty of water, as this can sometimes wash the bugs away. Aim for a minimum of three litres in a day

The Urinary Tract

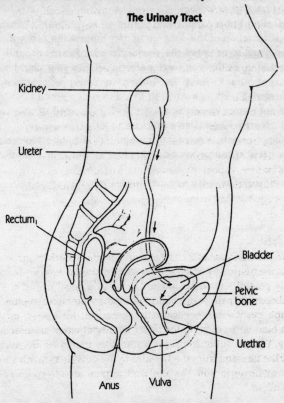

Kidney

Ureter

Rectum

Bladder

Pelvic bone

Urethra

Anus   Vulva

C

➤ sachets containing sodium or potassium citrate, available from chemists, make the urine less acid, and can help to relieve stinging and bladder irritation. Take one, three times a day, until symptoms go away – but not on a regular basis
➤ if symptoms persist for more than two days, if you have blood in your urine, if you have back pain or a high fever (suggesting a kidney infection) see your doctor straight away for antibiotic treatment
➤ keep warm and rest.

To prevent recurrent attacks
➤ Always empty your bladder either before, or preferably immediately after, making love.
➤ Wipe yourself from front to back after going to the toilet and if necessary, wash too, using warm water and cotton wool (again, wiping from front to back).
➤ Avoid using bubble baths and perfumed soaps, which can cause allergic irritation of the delicate tissues around the urethra.
➤ Never douche, or spray the shower head upwards around your vaginal area, as this can force bacteria up into your bladder.
➤ Recurrent attacks may be linked to using a contraceptive diaphragm. Consider switching to a different method.
➤ Make sure your vagina is always well lubricated during sex to avoid excess friction. Use a lubricating jelly if necessary.
➤ In older women, oestrogen cream, or hormone-replacement therapy (HRT) can prevent dryness and inflammation around the urethra.
➤ Drink a small glass of cranberry juice every day.

DANDRUFF

The white flakes of dandruff are dead cells, which are shed in excessive amounts from the surface of the scalp. In most cases an infection by the fungus, Pityrosporum, is to blame. This can either affect just a small area of the scalp, or in more severe cases, the whole of the scalp is covered in thick scales, which may be itchy. Mild dandruff may also be triggered by poor diet, for example, eating excess sugary products.

Self-help
➤ Shampoos containing tar, such as Polytar, or containing selenium sulphide may help mild cases. They should be used twice a week. Tea tree oil shampoo can be an effective natural remedy.
➤ Shampoo containing the anti-fungal ketoconazole (such as Nizoral) can be very effective, even for severe cases. It should be used twice a week for a month.
➤ Make sure you have a balanced, healthy diet with daily fruit, vegetables and wholegrains, and a low intake of sugar, tea, coffee and alcohol.

If self-help measures don't help, then see your GP. Occasionally a flaky scalp can be caused by eczema (see page 60) or psoriasis (see page 148).

DEPRESSION

It's normal to feel sad from time to time – it's part and parcel of a varied life. Depression is much more than this. It's a surprisingly common genuine mental illness, especially in women, who are affected twice as often as men. Symptoms vary in different people and according to the severity of the illness, but they can include:
➤ feeling low all the time, with bouts of crying for no good reason- feeling irritable and anxious
➤ loss of interest in hobbies or friends
➤ no energy. A common sign of depression is feeling tired all the time

D

> sleep disturbances. Sometimes this can be sleeping all the time, but waking early in the morning and not being able to get back to sleep again is more common
> a changed appetite, usually smaller, with weight loss
> low self-esteem – ' I'm no good for anybody or anything'
> in severe cases, life just doesn't seem worth living.

Depression is a major cause of attempts at, and success of, committing suicide.

Sometimes, depression can occur for an obvious reason, such as the death of a close friend or relative. In most of these cases there is a spontaneous recovery. But symptoms that persist for months on end, with no sign of any light at the end of the tunnel, should not be assumed to be normal. In many other cases, depression occurs out of the blue, for no apparent reason at all. Sometimes there can be a hidden underlying medical reason, such as an underactive thyroid, or it may be triggered by a nasty viral illness. Hormonal changes may also be to blame, such as at the time of the menopause, or after the birth of a baby.

Many cases of depression go unrecognised and untreated. Women seem reluctant to admit how they really feel, often for fear of being labelled as having a mental illness, or that everyone else will think they are going mad.

Self-help
The best way you can help yourself is to admit to yourself, and to others, how you really feel. Sometimes just talking about it to friends helps, but better still is to seek assistance from a person with training, either your doctor or a counsellor. Depression is nothing to be ashamed of, and if only more people would admit to it, the illness would be far better accepted. Struggling on, thinking that life will get better, is not the answer!

You can also help yourself by:

> keeping active. Exercise is good for the mind as well as the body, and can sometimes help to distract your thoughts away from things that may be troubling you
> eating sensible foods, such as pasta, and fresh fruit and vegetables. It's easy to lose weight and go short on essential vitamins if you've lost your appetite – so make sure the little that you do eat is as nutritious as possible
> don't be tempted to drown your sorrows in alcohol – it's only adding one problem on top of another, and will make you even more depressed.

D

Help from your doctor
Counselling or psychotherapy can be useful when depression is caused by specific events, or if it is part of an underlying personality problem. Counselling can either be done on a one-to-one basis, or as part of a group. Either way, your GP can refer you for expert help.

Anti-depressant drugs are highly effective, and unlike tranquillizers, they are not addictive. The most common types used are the tricyclics, which include dothiepin and amitriptilene, and a group of drugs known as SSRIs (serotonin re-uptake inhibitors) which include fluoxetine (or Prozac). Treatment is best continued until you've felt 'normal', and not depressed, for at least three months. Your GP can also arrange a referral to a hospital psychiatrist, but this is only necessary for very severe cases that don't respond to other treatments.

D AND C

This stands for dilatation and curettage. It's an operation to widen the neck of the womb, which enables the womb lining to be gently scraped out. It used to be done frequently as part of the investigation and treatment of period problems. However, new techniques, particularly vaginal ultrasound, and fine needle aspiration of the womb lining, mean that a D and C is rapidly becoming a rare operation. Fine needle aspiration is when the doctor removes a small portion of the womb lining for analysis, using a special fine needle and syringe. The main reason for a D and C now is to investigate bleeding after the menopause, and to remove polyps from the womb. It's usually done under general anaesthetic, but an overnight stay in hospital isn't normally required.

DIABETES

This is an illness in which there is a high level of glucose (sugar) in the bloodstream. This is caused by a shortage in the production of the hormone insulin from the pancreas. Insulin is vital for helping the sugar in the blood to move into other body cells, to be used as an energy source.
There are two main types of diabetes.
➤ The most severe form occurs when there is little, or no, insulin produced, because the secreting cells have been destroyed by the body's own immune system. This type, also known as type 1,

can occur at any age, but it tends to start in young people, especially children and teenagers. Approximately 60,000 people are affected with type 1 diabetes in the UK.

➤ The second type, of type II, occurs mainly in people over forty. Insulin is produced, but in amounts that are too small to adequately control the blood sugar level, especially in people who are overweight, or eat a diet high in sugar and carbohydrate. It is ten times more common than type 1 – affecting 600,000 people in the UK.

Diabetes can run in families. It can also be caused by some drugs, especially steroids, and may also occur during pregnancy – a condition called gestational diabetes. In these cases, once the baby is born, blood sugar levels tend to return to normal levels, but mothers who have developed this type of diabetes are at increased risk of becoming permanently diabetic later in life.

Symptoms

The high blood sugar levels that occur in diabetics can cause:

➤ the passage of large amounts of urine, which in turn can lead to increased thirst
➤ weakness and tiredness
➤ frequent infections. In women, recurrent bouts of thrush and cystitis are a commen problem.

If the blood sugar levels becomes extremely high (hyperglycaemia), the breath smells strangely acidic, and there may be mental confusion, and eventually coma. Though type 1 diabetes always causes noticeable symptoms, type II may only cause vague symptoms, such as tiredness, and remain undiagnosed for years.

Diabetes can cause more long-term serious health problems, especially in people who have either not been treated, or where despite treatment, the blood sugar level has remained high. These health problems include:

➤ thickening of the lining of the arteries, or atherosclerosis
➤ high blood pressure
➤ heart disease
➤ kidney damage, which may eventually lead to kidney failure
➤ nerve damage
➤ damage to the retina, the light-sensitive membrane in the back of the eye, which can eventually cause blindness. There is also an increased risk of cataracts.

D

Treatment

There are three main types of treatment.

❶ Many type II diabetics, especially those who are overweight, can control their blood sugar by diet alone. By losing weight and eating less sugars and carbohydrate, the blood sugar level often returns to normal.

❷ Where diet alone is insufficient, drugs can be used which boost the production of insulin from the pancreas.

❸ Type 1 diabetics require treatment with insulin, which has to be injected directly into the body tissues, usually into the lower abdomen, or the leg. There are two main types of insulin available. The most common type used is a genetically-engineered version of human insulin manufactured in laboratories. However, some patients prefer to use animal insulin, usually obtained from pigs.

Insulins also vary in the length of time they work inside the body. Some only need to be given once or twice a day, others up to four times a day. Most diabetics use a combination of short- and long-acting varieties to give good control of their blood sugar level. An excess of insulin, either due to too high a dose, or not eating enough food, can lead to a dangerous fall in the blood sugar level, a condition known as hypoglycaemia. The first symptoms of this are usually confusion, weakness, and pale, clammy, sweaty skin. If it is not treated promptly by eating glucose, it can rapidly lead to coma and sometimes even death. As a precaution, all insulin-dependent diabetics should carry some glucose tablets with them at all times.

For long-term control, all diabetics should check their own blood sugar levels on a regular basis. This can be done using a tiny droplet of blood on a special small test strip. In addition, all diabetics should have a regular check-up, at least once a year, by a specially trained nurse or doctor.

DIARRHOEA

This is the frequent passage of loose or watery motions. Acute, short-lived attacks lasting less than twelve hours are commonly due to eating contaminated food or water. Recurrent bouts of diarrhoea can be caused by anxiety and stress, and can be a sign of irritable bowel syndrome (see page 116).

Diarrhoea can also be caused by food intolerance, an over-active thyroid gland, and less commonly, by inflammation in the lining of the bowel. Occasionally recurrent diarrhoea can be a symptom of bowel cancer.

Self-help
During an acute attack:
➤ prevent dehydration by drinking plenty of water. Add a pinch of salt to each small glassful, to replace that lost from the body, together with a teaspoonful of sugar for energy. Or buy special fluid replacement sachets from the chemist, such as Rehydrat or Diorylyte
➤ stop eating solid food for at least twelve hours and avoid anything containing milk, until the diarrhoea subsides
➤ if you have to travel, loperamide capsules, available from chemists, are usually very effective at stopping diarrhoea on a temporary basis.

Help from your doctor
You should see a doctor for investigations if you have:
➤ blood in your motions
➤ diarrhoea for more than a week
➤ repeated bouts of diarrhoea, especially coupled with stomach pains.

DIGESTIVE PROBLEMS

Many of the problems that arise in the upper part of the digestive tract are due in part to the strongly acidic juices secreted by the stomach, that are essential for food digestion.

HEARTBURN

This is caused by acid leaking back up from the stomach into the oesophagus, the food pipe that travels from the mouth to the stomach. It causes a burning sensation in the chest, usually behind the breast bone, but the discomfort may reach as far as the mouth, together with a sour acid taste. Repeated bouts of heartburn can lead to inflammation in the delicate lining of the oesophagus (oesophagitis).

The acid reflux occurs because of a weakness in the sphincter muscle at the top of the stomach. In women especially, it can also be due to a hiatus hernia, in which the top portion of the stomach slides up into the chest.

Self-help for heartburn
➤ Eat slowly, and avoid spicy, fatty foods and excessive amounts of alcohol or caffeine, which can irritate the oesophagus.

➤ Don't lie down for at least two hours or more after eating.
➤ Excess body fat collects inside, as well as on the outside, of your waistline, and can put extra pressure on the stomach. Getting your weight back to normal can often cure heartburn alone!
➤ Special antacids containing alginates, which are available from chemists, act as a barrier and prevent acid reflux.
➤ Medicines that reduce the secretion of acid, such as cimetidine and ranitidine, can be very effective at preventing and treating heartburn, and are available directly from chemists.

D

Help from your doctor
You should see a doctor if you have persistent symptoms. A gastroscopy – when the oesophagus and stomach are examined directly through a flexible telescope – can rule out a serious cause.

The drug Omeprazole, only available on prescription, reduces acid secretion and is highly effective for heartburn and oesophagitis.

INDIGESTION
This can vary from a feeling of fullness, to severe discomfort, to shooting pains, usually in the top of the abdomen, especially on the left side. In severe cases, it can easily be mistaken for a heart attack.

Women vary in their susceptibility to indigestion. Whilst some lucky ones can eat or drink anything without any problems, for others the slightest dietary indiscretion can lead to hours of discomfort afterwards. Though this is partly related to the amount of acid secreted by the stomach, there is increasing evidence that a stomach infection with the bacteria Helicobacter Pylori (H.Pylori) can make a person much more susceptible to inflammation of the stomach, stomach ulcers and also stomach cancer later in life.

Prevention
➤ Eat slowly, sitting down. Don't feel you have to clear your plate – stop when you're full.
➤ Keeping your mouth closed when you're eating actually has more to it than good manners – it prevents you swallowing excessive amounts of air, which can cause indigestion.
➤ Avoid gassy drinks, such as coke, fizzy water, or spirits mixed with carbonated mixers. Have still water, fruit juice (but not orange juice which is very acidic and can trigger indigestion) or still wine instead.

➤ Avoid very hot or spicy foods, and large amounts of alcohol, which can irritate the stomach lining. Stop smoking too, as this increases stomach acid production.

D

Self-help
➤ A good home-made remedy is half a teaspoonful of bicarbonate of soda, mixed in half a glass of warm water, with a drop of peppermint oil.
➤ Numerous medicines are available from chemists that help to neutralize stomach acid. Liquid versions are usually more effective than tablets.
➤ Most effective of all are tablets that actually reduce acid secretion, such as cimetidine or ranitidine. They are however, much more expensive than other remedies.

Help from your doctor
➤ Anyone suffering repeated bouts of pain or discomfort should see a doctor to rule out a more serious cause, such as stomach inflammation (gastritis) or an ulcer.
➤ Infection with H. Pylori can now be simply and quickly diagnosed with either a breath or blood test. Treating the infection with a combination of antibiotics, together with a drug that reduces acid secretion, can cure many cases of chronic indigestion and recurrent ulcers.
➤ Occasionally, indigestion can be a side effect of prescribed medicines. Check with your doctor.

DISCHARGE

Many women assume that a vaginal discharge means there is an infection present. This is quite wrong. Though infections can cause a discharge, some of the more serious ones often don't. A discharge is often commonly the sign of either mild inflammation or an allergy, or can even just be a natural fertility signal! The vagina is normally kept moist by mucus and fluid secreted by the glands at the vaginal entrance and from the cervix. This fluid is rich in 'good' bacteria, known as lactobacilli, which make the vaginal secretions acid and help to protect the vagina from infections.

Around the time of ovulation, there's an increase in the secretion of cervical mucus, which can appear as clear, sticky discharge. This usually starts a few days before ovulation, and stops the day after the egg has been released. It's a useful indicator of the most fertile

D

VAGINAL DISCHARGE – QUICK GUIDE

Discharge	Likely cause	Action
Clear, sticky, no smell.	Increased oestrogen. Normal for a few days before ovulation. Also common in pill users.	None needed unless persistent and a nuisance. Changing pill may help.
Creamy white, thick, musty smell, soreness and itching.	Thrush	Anti-fungal cream and pessaries. See a doctor if persists.
Slight creamy, fishy smell.	Gardnerella	Occasionally gets better on its own. If present for more than a few days see a doctor for antibiotics.
Green, frothy, itchy and sore.	Trichomonas	See a doctor for antibiotics.
Slight green or cream, no noticeable smell.	Could be chlamydia or gonorrhoea.	See a doctor for tests and treatment.
Brown staining	Caused by old blood.	See a doctor to identify the cause.
Profuse, watery greeny, with foul smell.	Retained tampon or contraceptive.	Check! See a doctor if you can't find a cause, or if it's stuck.
Slight watery or green, soreness or irritation, in older women.	Inflammation due to lack of oestrogen.	See a doctor for proper diagnosis, and treatment with oestrogen cream or HRT.

time of the month – for either having intercourse or using additional contraceptive precautions, depending on whether you want to get pregnant or not!

The oestrogen in the combined contraceptive pill and higher dose hormone-replacement therapy (HRT) preparations can cause an increase in the natural vaginal secretions in some women. It's also normal to have an increased clear, slightly sticky discharge during sexual arousal. Though these natural discharges may give a slight yellow stain on underwear, there should be no itching, and no smell.

Occasionally a persistent clear, or slightly yellow coloured sticky discharge can be due to a cervical erosion (see page 37). Though this is quite harmless, it can be a nuisance, and if you find you always have staining on your pants, or always have to wear a pad, then you should see a doctor for an internal examination (don't worry, this shouldn't hurt!)

The other common non-infectious cause of a discharge is an allergic reaction inside the vagina. Perfumed bubble baths, soaps, or vaginal deodorants are common culprits, but contraceptives such as jellies, foams or the rubber in caps and condoms may also be to blame. The vagina may just feel uncomfortable, or itchy, or sore, and there may be a creamy discharge, but again, it shouldn't smell.

INFECTIONS

The commonest cause of an itchy discharge is thrush (see page 164). This discharge is usually thick, sometimes lumpy, creamy white or yellow, and has a slight musty smell. Thrush often also causes noticeable red swelling of the tissues around the vagina. Thrush is usually a women's problem (athough it is occasionally sexually transmitted), and effective treatment is available directly from chemists.

The other cause of an itchy discharge is trichomonas vaginalis or TV, (see page 169). This tends to cause a watery, or frothy green, or yellow discharge. Unlike thrush, this is usually sexually transmitted, and effective treatment (the antibiotic Metronidazole) is available only on prescription.

A creamy or watery discharge with a noticeable fishy smell is most likely to be due to gardnerella vaginalis (see page 85). Like TV, this needs treatment with Metronidazole, available only on prescription.

Rather surprisingly, the more serious sexually transmitted infections, gonorrhoea and chlamydia, often don't cause a noticeable discharge. Occasionally they cause a slight cream or green discharge, but unlike thrush or TV, there's no itching.

Any brown discoloration in a discharge is a sign of old, slightly dried blood. Unless it occurs at either the beginning or end of a period, this should always be investigated by a doctor.

D

Self-help

In some cases, it's possible to effectively treat discharge yourself. See the chart (page 57), but don't hesitate to see a doctor if you're not sure of the cause, or if self-treatment doesn't work. Don't carry on buying several different medicines from the chemist, see a doctor for proper tests and treatment. You can either go to your GP, or alternatively, you can go to your local hospital department of Genito-Urinary medicine. You don't need a referral letter. They can do tests on the spot, and can often give an accurate instant diagnosis.

If you're prone to a discharge, avoid using perfumed soaps and don't add anything to your bath water. Perfumed bubble baths and antiseptics such as Dettol should be avoided especially, and never, ever douche. Avoid perfumed contraceptive creams and gels and use hypo-allergic brands instead. Special hypo-allergic condoms are also available.

DOUCHING

The abundant natural secretions inside the vagina act not only as a remarkably efficient self-cleansing mechanism, but also anti-bacterial and help to protect the vagina from infection. Washing them away by swooshing or spraying water up into the vagina does nothing but harm. Adding chemicals to the water, such as soaps or antiseptics, is a good recipe for either vaginal inflammation or an infection!

Douching after unprotected intercourse won't help prevent a pregnancy, and if you've already got a vaginal infection it will make it worse, not better. So leave douching where it belongs – in the history books!

E

ECTOPIC PREGNANCY

This is a pregnancy which for unknown reasons develops anywhere outside the womb. The most common site is inside one of the Fallopian tubes. Rarely do ectopics occur in an ovary, or further afield in the abdominal cavity. About one in 200 pregnancies in this country is an ectopic. As the pregnancy grows, the lining of the tube is damaged and can rupture, causing severe, heavy bleeding. If this isn't treated immediately, life-threatening heavy bleeding can occur. Ectopic pregnancies still kill seven women in the UK each year.

Ectopics can occur in any woman, but some are more at risk. These include women with damaged tubes, either as a result of pelvic infection, or previous tubal surgery, (or occasionally after sterilization) women who fall pregnant whilst using a coil, or the progesterone-only pill, and women who have had a previous ectopic.

The first signs of an ectopic usually occur about two weeks after the missed period, and are light bleeding from the vagina, and lower abdominal pain. Occasionally, the first sign is more dramatic, with severe abdominal pain (from internal bleeding), and shock.

Anyone with even vague signs of an ectopic should see a doctor straight away. Diagnosis is by ultrasound (see page 170), together with a laparoscopy if necessary (see page 118).

Once an ectopic is confirmed, it's essential to remove the foetus to prevent further bleeding. In the early stages of a pregnancy, this can often be done without damaging the Fallopian tube, but in more advanced cases, removal of part of the tube may be necessary.

Sadly, having an ectopic inevitably means losing the baby. As yet, no doctor has ever succeeded in transferring a baby to a womb.

ECZEMA

This is inflamed, scaly, itchy skin. There are two main types. Atopic eczema is due to an over reaction of the body's own immune system, that can be inherited, and is often linked with other allergic problems, such as asthma and hayfever. Common areas affected include the backs of the knees, the wrists and the face.

Contact eczema, or dermatitis, is caused by direct irritation of the skin. Common triggers are household cleaners and detergents, perfumes, and nickel – found in a lot of jewellery and jeans studs.

Self-help
➤ Preventing dryness is essential. Use an unperfumed moistuizing cream on all dry areas at least twice a day.
➤ Avoid bubble baths and soap – use special unperfumed moisturizing bath oils instead, such as Balneum.
➤ Don't wear wool or other itchy fabrics next to your skin. Pure cotton is best, as this allows the skin to breathe.
➤ Wear cotton-lined rubber gloves for all household chores.
➤ Avoid jewellery containing nickel. Wear pure silver or gold instead, or coat the back of earring or earstuds with clear nail varnish.
➤ 1 percent hydrocortisone cream (available from chemists) can help to relieve itching and soreness. But don't use it on your face, and for no more than two weeks elsewhere.

Help from your doctor
➤ Larger quantities of emollients and bath oils are cheaper via a prescription.
➤ Stronger steroid creams, which are very effective, are only available on prescription, but they must be used very carefully, to avoid skin damage.
➤ If necessary, your doctor can refer you for skin testing to try and identify the cause of contact dermatitis.

EMERGENCY CONTRACEPTION

This is a way of preventing a pregnancy after unprotected sex. Its other name, the 'morning-after' contraception, is misleading and inaccurate, as emergency contraception can be effective even after a delay of several days.

Emergency contraception is available from most GPs and all family planning clinics.

There are two methods available.
❶ The Pill method can be used up to seventy-two hours (three days) after unprotected sex. It involves taking two sets of two high-dose ordinary contraceptive pills, twelve hours apart. Almost any woman can use this method, even older women who smoke, and who shouldn't normally take the Pill. The most common side-

effect is nausea, and occasional vomiting, but these are not common. The Pill method is very effective, but women who've taken it still do become pregnant. This is more likely if unprotected sex has occurred mid-way between periods, around the time of ovulation. But if a pregnancy does occur, there's no evidence that the 'morning-after' Pill is dangerous to the baby. The Pill method is only effective for sex that's taken place in the previous three days. If you have unprotected sex again, after you've taken the pills, you need to take another lot.

❷ The second method involves having a coil, or intra-uterine contraceptiver device (IUCD) fitted. This works by preventing implantation if an egg is fertilized. This method is effective if the coil is inserted up to five days after the estimated date of ovulation. For a women with a twenty-eight day monthly cycle, ovulation occurs around day fourteen, (counting the first day of bleeding as day one), which means that a coil can be inserted effectively up to day nineteen – no matter when or how often unprotected sex has taken place. This timing can be difficult for many women to calculate – see your GP or practice nurse for more help if you need to. The coil can be left in place to provide future contraception, or alternatively, it can be removed during the next period. Any women can be fitted with a coil, although it's best avoided if there's any evidence of a vaginal infection that might cause pelvic inflammatory disease (PID). Women who've never been pregnant do sometimes find the fitting a bit uncomfortable, but overall this is a better option than risking an unwanted pregnancy.

ENDOMETRIOSIS

This is a condition affecting at least 10 percent of women, in which tissue like that which is lining the womb is found elsewhere in the body. The most common sites are in the pelvis, the ovaries, around the Fallopian tubes, and on the ligaments that support the womb. But endometriosis can be found anywhere, such as in the bowel, or even in the tummy button (though this is much more rare). This tissue changes throughout the monthly cycle just like the womb lining. In particular it thickens, and then bleeds at period time. The blood irritates the delicate pelvic organs, causing inflammation, scarring and pain. In the ovaries, blood filled cysts can form (known as chocolate cysts).

The exact cause for endometriosis is not known, but the most popular theory is that it results from 'retrograde menstruation' – that is, bleeding backwards, up the Fallopian tubes at period time.

Some women with fertility problems are found, during investigations, to have endometriosis. In many cases, this is a mysterious link, as the Fallopian tubes are undamaged and ovulation occurs as normal. Having endometriosis certainly does not mean you are bound to have difficulty getting pregnant.

Symptoms

The most common symptom is pain, which builds up for a few days before each period, and is then at its worst during the first few days of bleeding. The pain can be very severe, and even strong prescription painkillers may be ineffective at giving relief. Pain often also occurs during and after intercourse, and during a pelvic examination by a doctor.

Other symptoms can include lower back pain, pain passing urine, and a dull ache in the pelvis which never really goes away. Interestingly, however, some women having pelvic surgery for other reasons are found to have endometriosis which has apparently caused no symptoms at all.

The diagnosis can be suspected from symptoms and a pelvic examination (but it is often mistaken for pelvic inflammatory disease PID). A pelvic ultrasound scan may reveal swellings on the tubes or ovaries that make the diagnosis likely, but the only way that endometriosis can be properly confirmed is by a laparoscopy (see page 118), when a gynaecologist can actually see the deposits. Women with severe symptoms may be found to have tiny areas affected, while women who are found to have large deposits may have only mild symptoms. It's an unpredictable disease.

Treatment

This depends on the severity of the symptoms. It usually involves hormone treatment of some sort, but in more severe cases surgery may also be required (or may be the option chosen).

The aim of hormone treatment is to stop the cyclical build-up and shedding of both the womb lining and endometriotic tissue. Treatment needs to be continued for at least six months, and sometimes much longer. For the best effect, periods should stop completely during this time. Some gynaecologists recommend a further laparoscopy after treatment to check if any endometriosis still remains.

In mild cases, progesterone tablets, or the combined oral contraceptive pill, taken continuously, may be helpful. More effective treatments include:

➤ Danazol – a well-tried drug that reduces secretion of the hormones from the pituitary gland which stimulate the ovaries. Unfortunately, side effects are common, and more likely at the higher, more effective doses, and can include weight gain, oily skin and acne, excess body hair, nausea and dizziness

➤ Gestrinone – similar to danazol, with similar side effects, but some women find it suits them better. It is only taken twice a week

➤ Buserelin and Goserelin – powerful (and expensive!) drugs that completely switch off production in the pituitary gland of the hormones that stimulate ovarian activity. Oestrogen production from the ovary falls dramatically, and this can commonly cause menopause-like symptoms such as hot flushes, sweats, vaginal dryness and a decreased libido.

Surgical treatments are best reserved for severe cases that do not respond to treatment with drugs, or for women who are unable to tolerate the side-effects. Small patches of endometriosis can be destroyed by heat, using either cautery or a laser. This is performed via a laparoscope. Endometriotic ovarian cysts can be removed, and the rest of the ovary left intact. If endometriosis is severe, and there is a lot of scarring, the best treatment is often to remove the affected organs. This may mean a hysterectomy, together with removal of both the ovaries and Fallopian tubes. Though this sounds drastic, it can give welcome relief to women who have suffered many years of severe pain. Young women under forty-five who have had both their ovaries removed should have hormone-replacement therapy (HRT) to prevent osteoporosis and heart disease. However, because the hormones in HRT can stimulate the growth of endometriosis, it's best to wait at least six months after any surgery to allow any residual endometriosis to completely disappear.

EROSION
(see Cervix page 37.)

EXERCISE
Exercise helps almost everything in your body work better – and that includes your mind!

There are three main types of exercise.

❶ Aerobic exercise – such as jogging, brisk walking, swimming or cycling – increases the heart rate and the body's need for oxygen. This type of exercise is good for the heart, making it work more efficiently, and can also help to prevent high blood pressure. This type of exercise can also boost levels of HDL cholesterol, which also helps to protect against heart disease.

❷ Weight-bearing exercise includes tennis, walking, running, stair climbing and weight training. This type of exercise can help to increase bone mass, and prevent osteoporosis.

❸ Stretching exercises, which includes swimming, increase joint flexibility and muscle tone, and also help to prevent injuries from other types of more vigorous exercise.

In addition to all these benefits, regular exercise is essential for a well-toned figure, and can be an invaluable aid in weight control. By increasing the production of endorphins and enkephalins, the body's own 'happy hormones', it can also be a natural mood lifter. It's a good remedy for stress, and can help to prevent depression.

There's no firm rule about how much exercise is necessary for good health. Although some experts have said that you need twenty minutes, three times a week, at a level that makes you slightly puffed, other doctors say that thirty minutes of moderate activity every day is better. What is certain is that any exercise is better than none at all, and that generally the more you do, the greater the benefits for your body and soul!

How to take more exercise

There are two ways:

❶ The first, and most important, is to increase your daily activity levels. Do this by:
  ➤ altering the way you travel to work, or when you visit friends. Either walk, or cycle, or if you take public transport, walk to the next stop along, rather than the one outside your front door
  ➤ walking upstairs rather than using the escalator or lift
  ➤ turning off the TV in the evenings and weekends, and involving the whole family in an activity, such as a game of football, or going for a long walk.

❷ The second way is to take up a sport – the range is so great now that anyone, of any age, can enjoy a new hobby. Choose something which you are likely to enjoy, and which fits in with your lifestyle. If you're unsure about your fitness, see your GP first for a check-up. You should also ask for advice if you've ever had a heart condition or chest trouble; if you're troubled by arthritis or joint pains; if you're diabetic; or if you're recovering from an illness or operation.

When you're taking up a new sport, always start gently, and gradually increase the amount you do, week by week. To avoid injury, it's important to warm up your muscles first with a few gentle bends and stretches.

Don't exercise straight after a meal – it's a good recipe for indigestion. Always wait for at least an hour. Don't exercise if you have a heavy cold or if you're unwell. Wait until you feel better, and then start slowly.

E

EYE PROBLEMS

Left alone, the delicate tissues of the eyes are remarkably good at looking after themselves but wearing eye make-up means that women are more prone to eye problems than men.

CONJUNCTIVITIS

This is an inflammation of the lining of the eye. It causes soreness and a gritty feeling in the front of the eye. It can be caused by an allergic reaction, most commonly to pollen in the hay fever season, but reactions to eye creams and make-up are also quite common. Allergic reactions may only affect one eye, but usually both are red and inflamed. Drops containing sodium cromoglycate (available from chemists) can ease allergic conjunctivitis, usually within hours.

Conjunctivitis can also be caused by an infection with either viruses or bacteria. It's more common in people who wear contact lenses and usually only one eye is affected. Viral conjunctivitis causes intense redness, and a profuse watery discharge. Bacterial conjunctivitis causes a thick pus-like discharge, and can be treated with antibiotic drops, available on prescription from your GP.

STYES

These are caused by an infection in an eyelash follicle, leading to a sore, red swelling on the eyelid. They usually get better on their own, but if they persist for more than a week, or if the swelling spreads, then treatment with antibiotic ointment (from your GP) may be helpful.

SWOLLEN, ITCHY EYELIDS

These are usually caused by an allergic reaction. Finding the cause can be very difficult. Although the culprit may be something that's been in direct contact with the eyes, foods such as peanuts or strawberries are a common cause. The swelling can often be eased by taking an anti-histamine, and applying a very weak hydrocortisone cream.

Preventing eye problems
➤ Wear dark sunglasses in bright sunlight. As well as making vision more comfortable, this can also help to protect your eyes from ultra-violet rays, which can cause cataracts.
➤ Only use light creams around the eyes that are specifically designed for that area. Using a heavy face cream can cause puffiness.
➤ Avoid wearing kohl or eyeliner on the inside of the lashes as small flakes can easily fall into the eye and cause irritation.
➤ Mascara and liquid eyeliner can easily become contaminated. If you get an eye infection, throw them away and buy new ones.
➤ If you work with a VDU, take a break from the screen at least once every two hours. This can help to prevent tired, dry eyes and eye strain.
➤ Dark rings can be a sign of stress and lost sleep!

E

FALLOPIAN TUBES

Every women normally has two tiny tubes, about 7.5cm long, that extend outwards from the top corners of the womb where the ovaries are. Each tube widens at its free end, which lies close to an ovary.

The Fallopian tubes are a very important part of a woman's reproductive system. It's where an egg and sperm usually meet, and where fertilization takes place. Tiny hairs waft the developing embryo down towards the womb. Occasionally, this transport system fails, and the embryo becomes lodged in the tube and becomes an ectopic pregnancy (see page 60). Damaged or blocked Fallopian tubes are a common cause of infertility. The most common reason for this is scarring following infection (which accounts for 15 percent of infertility cases), but damage from endometriosis, or previous pelvic surgery can also be to blame. Any scarring inside the tube also increases the risk of an ectopic.

Though tubal surgery is sometimes performed to remove the scarred part of a tube, pregnancy rates afterwards are disappointing. Better results are usually obtained from IVF (see page 112), and in many centres tubal surgery has been abandoned apart from correcting very minor damage.

FAMILY PLANNING

The ever-increasing range of family planning methods available today really does mean that most couples can enjoy a fulfilling sexual relationship without risking an unwanted pregnancy.

However, when you're choosing a method, it's important to be realistic. The ideal contraceptive is one that's 100 percent reliable, with no side-effects and sadly, it still doesn't exist. Every single method available has drawbacks – either in terms of side-effects, or in terms of reliability. You need to decide what is most important for you. But remember, apart from sterilization, no method is permanent, and you may change your mind. So, if you find one particular method isn't suitable, try something else. It's vital you find a method that suits your circumstances and lifestyle now.

Where to go
There are two main sources. Most GPs supply basic methods, such as the Pill, but not all are trained at fitting coils and caps – although there may be another doctor or nurse at your local practice who can help instead. Tell the receptionist what you want, so that she can give you an appropriate appointment.

You are also free to see another GP, outside your practice, for Family Planning Services only. If you choose this option it should not affect your relationship with your regular GP. Alternatively, you can go to a Family Planning Clinic run by your local Health Authority. Here you should find expertise in all methods, but opening times may be restricted. All Family Planning in this country should be provided free of charge.

F

HORMONAL METHODS
These include the combined pill (often known as simply 'the Pill'); the progesterone-only pill (often known as the 'mini-Pill'); injectables and implants; and the new progesterone-containing coil, Mirena.

In general, hormonal methods are more effective than barrier methods, but have more side-effects. They also have the disadvantage that they offer little protection against sexually transmitted infections.

THE COMBINED PILL
This contains two hormones, oestrogen and progesterone, and it works by preventing the monthly release of an egg from the ovaries. It also alters the lining of the womb, preventing implantation in the unlikely event of fertilization of an egg taking place.

It's usually taken for three weeks, followed by a seven day break, when a light, pill-withdrawal bleed occurs.

Advantages
➤ It's very effective, with less than a 1 percent failure rate.
➤ It gives light, regular periods, which are often much less painful than before.
➤ By reducing blood loss, it can help to prevent anaemia.
➤ It can reduce the risk of benign breast disease and cyclical breast pain.
➤ It can reduce pre-menstrual syndrome (PMS).
➤ It can help to protect against cancer of the ovaries and of the womb.
➤ It can be taken by many women right up to the menopause.
➤ It allows spontaneous sex, with no fiddling about, and no mess!

Disadvantages
➤ It's not suitable for women with certain medical conditions including: heart disease; high blood pressure; liver disease; clotting problems; some types of migraine; gallstones; and any cancer that's stimulated by oestrogen.
➤ Prolonged use of the Pill at a young age probably increases the risk of breast cancer. Women with a strong family history of breast cancer should avoid this method.
➤ Women who smoke should stop the Pill at thirty-five. Smokers who are overweight should stop even earlier.
➤ It's not suitable for breast-feeding mums.
➤ Side-effects can be a worry, and a nuisance. The Pill can increase the risk, very slightly, of strokes, heart attacks, and clots in veins. Minor side-effects can include nausea, tender breasts, weight gain, acne, headaches and fluid retention. Many of these problems can be solved by switching brands (see below).
➤ It needs to be taken reliably, every day, to be effective. (For instructions about missed pills, see below.)
➤ Its effect can be reduced by some drugs, especially antibiotics.

Choosing a Pill
There are more than twenty-five different brands of combined pill available. Though they all contain the same oestrogen (ethinyl oestradiol), strengths vary between 20–50mcg. The most commonly prescribed pills contain 30mcg or 35mcg. Those containing higher doses are more likely to give side effects such as bloating, weight gain and nausea, particularly in the first few months. Switching to lower dose formulation may help. There are two ultra-low dose formulations – Loestrin 20 and Mercilon, that contain only 20mcg oestrogen. Unfortunately, breakthrough bleeding is slightly more common with these, and they may be slightly less effective as contraceptives (especially if a pill is accidently missed).

Combined pills can contain one of five different types of progesterone or progestogen. Side-effects from the progesterone component can include acne, weight gain and pre-menstrual tension (PMT) type symptoms. If these are a problem, then try switching to a brand with a different, or lower levels of progesterone. Pills containing desogestrel (such as Marvelon and Mercilon) and gestodene (such as Femodene) have a slightly increased risk of causing venous thrombosis (a blood clot in a vein) compared to other progestogens, so these pills are probably best reserved as a second choice when others don't suit.

Bi-phasic (such as Bi-novum) and tri-phasic pills (such as Trinordial and Tri-novum) contain differing amounts of hormones at different stages of the Pill cycle. They are more complicated to take (especially if you want to delay your period), but they can be useful for women who suffer breakthrough bleeding with other brands.

Your GP or Family Planning Doctor should be able to help you. What's important is that there is a wide choice of different pills available, and it's normally possible to find a brand that suits most women. Try and stick to a brand for a least three months, as many side-effects do settle down, but then if you're still having problems, see your doctor.

F

Missed pills
To be effective, apart from the seven day break, each pill should be taken within thirty-six hours of the previous pill. This means that you don't have to take the Pill at the same time each day – you have twelve hours grace – though obviously it's best to get into a good daily routine if possible.

If more than thirty-six hours pass between pills, take the missed Pill as soon as possible. But you then need to use extra precautions for the next seven days – while you carry on taking your pills as usual. If there are less than seven pills left in the packet, go straight on to the next packet without a break. This will mean you don't have a period, but this doesn't matter. If you have sex without extra precautions in the week after a missed pill, see your doctor as soon as possible to discuss emergency contraception (see page 61).

Vomiting or severe diarrhoea can also affect pill absorption. Apply the 'missed Pill' rules until your tummy has settled.

THE PROGESTERONE-ONLY PILL
Also known as the POP, the mini-pill, or the everyday pill, this contains a small dose of just one hormone, progesterone. It works by thickening the mucus in the neck of the womb, making it impenetrable to sperm. It also thins the lining of the womb (making it more difficult for a fertilized egg to implant), and in a few women it stops ovulation. Unlike the combined pill, the POP must be taken every single day, without a break.

Advantages
➤ More effective than many barrier methods (but slightly less effective than the combined pill). With careful use it has a failure rate

of 1–2 percent. But larger women, please note – if you're over 70kg you should take two pills each day.

➤ Has fewer side effects than the combined pill.
➤ Can be used by many women who can't take the combined pill for medical reasons, including older women who smoke, and breast feeding mums.
➤ Can reduce period problems, including heavy bleeding, and PMT.
➤ By thickening the cervical mucus, it offers a little protection against pelvic inflammatory disease (PID).
➤ Like the combined pill, it allows hassle-free, spontaneous sex.

Disadvantages
➤ Has to be taken at the same time each day.
➤ Can cause erratic periods, and spotting or bleeding in-between periods.
➤ Some women have long gaps between periods. In fact, this tends to signify delayed ovulation, which means the Pill is working very well as a contraceptive!
➤ Side-effects can include headaches, greasy skin, acne, weight gain and occasionally, loss of libido.
➤ Can increase the risk of an ectopic pregnancy. Women who have had an ectopic should avoid using this method.

Choosing a Pill
There are only six different types available, containing four different progesterones. Two types, Noriday and Micronor, contain exactly the same active ingredient! If one pill is causing side-effects, it's always worth trying another brand.

Missed Pills
This is more of a problem with the POP than the combined pill. Each POP can only be taken up to three hours late – that's twenty-seven hours from the previous pill. After that, it counts as a missed pill, and you should use extra precautions for the following seven days, while you carry on taking your pill as normal. The same rules apply if you have vomiting or severe diarrhoea.

INJECTABLES AND IMPLANTS
These contain long-acting versions of the hormone progesterone. There are two injections available – Noristerat, which lasts two months, and Depo-Provera, which lasts three months. The implant

version, Norplant, consists of six rods that are inserted under the skin of the upper arm. It's effective for up to five years, when the rods should be removed. However, the rods can be removed much sooner than this if desired. They all work in a way similar to the progesterone-only pill, by thickening the mucus at the womb entrance to prevent sperm penetration. Like the POP, they also thin the lining of the womb. They differ from the POP in that they are more likely to stop ovulation – hence they are more effective contraceptives.

Injectables – advantages
➤ Very effective. Has a less than 1 percent failure rate.
➤ Long-lasting, and so suitable for women who have trouble taking pills regularly.
➤ Periods may become very light and in some women, they stop altogether. This can help women prone to anaemia from heavy periods.
➤ Allows hassle-free, spontaneous sex.

Injectables – disadvantages
➤ Can cause menstrual chaos with heavy, continued bleeding. This is more likely in the first few months of use.
➤ Can cause side-effects, such as weight gain, greasy skin, and acne.
➤ After several injections, there may be a delay of up to a year before fertility returns.
➤ Once it's in, it can't be taken out, or its effect reversed. Any unwanted effects may continue for three months or more.
➤ Some patients have difficulty remembering when their next injection is due.

Norplant – advantages
➤ Very effective, especially in the first year after insertion (less than 1 percent failure rate). In the subsequent years, the failure rate stays very low, at 1–2 percent, which is better than the POP.
➤ Often leads to very light, pain-free periods.
➤ Provides contraception for up to five years.
➤ Once the rods are removed, fertility returns within a few days.

Norplant – disadvantages
➤ Needs a local anaesthetic for insertion, and the arm can be uncomfortable and sore for several days afterwards.

➤ The insertion and removal cuts may leave small permanent scars.
➤ The rods can be difficult to remove.
➤ Periods may become very erratic, with variable flow (sometimes heavy, sometimes light).
➤ Side effects can include headaches, nausea, weight gain, acne and breast tenderness.

Norplant rods should always be inserted and removed by fully trained doctors who are experienced in the techniques involved. If you are considering Norplant please make sure that before the rods are inserted, you have full counselling and if possible, are given written information about any possible side-effects you may experience. Norplant is probably best reserved for women who've found other methods unsuitable.

THE PROGESTERONE INTRA-UTERINE SYSTEM (IUS) OR MIRENA

This is a revolutionary new type of coil that was launched in the UK in 1995, which had been well tried, tested and available in Europe for many years before this.

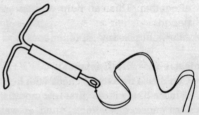

Unlike normal coils, which have copper around the stem, the Mirena has a core of the progesterone, levonorgestrel, around the stem. This adds to its contraceptive efficiency and vastly reduces problems from side-effects.

It works in several ways. The progesterone thickens the cervical mucus, preventing sperm penetration, and thins the lining of the womb, making it more difficult for a fertilized egg to implant. It also interferes with sperm transport through the womb. In many ways, the coil part just acts as a holder of the progesterone, but it adds to the contraceptive efficacy by additionally interfering with any sperm that do reach the womb.

Advantages
➤ It's incredibly effective. Its failure rate is lower than all the other methods, except possibly sterilization.
➤ Makes periods much lighter and shorter.
➤ It's usually easy to insert or remove, especially in women who have had children.
➤ Its effect can be reversed by simply removing the device.

➤ Provides hassle-free contraception, allowing spontaneous sex, for up to three years.
➤ Is suitable for nearly all women of all ages.

Disadvantages
➤ Light, erratic bleeding may occur in the first three months after insertion.
➤ Rarely, progesterone-related side-effects may occur, such as weight gain or acne.
➤ Insertion may be difficult and painful, and require a local anaesthetic for women who have never been pregnant.

Compared to the Pill, or an ordinary copper coil, Mirenas are expensive for the NHS (making some doctors reluctant to fit them). However, they are excellent contraceptives, and a welcome addition to the choice available. In future, Mirenas may well be used for purposes other than straight contraception, such as a treatment for heavy periods, or as the progesterone component of hormone-replacement therapy (HRT).

INTRA-UTERINE CONTRACEPTIVE DEVICES (IUCDs) OR COILS

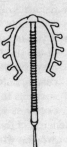

Coils are small pieces of plastic about 1.5.cm long, which have copper wire round around the stem. The versions used today are either shaped like a variant of a T, or an inverted U. The copper 7, a popular device in the past, is now obsolete.

All coils have to be carefully placed inside the womb cavity by a specially trained doctor or nurse. Each coil has either one or two thin nylon threads which are cut after insertion, so that a short length is left protruding out through the cervix and into the vagina. These threads should not interfere with intercourse in any way (if they do – see your doctor).

Coils work by interfering with the way sperm swim up through the womb, helping to prevent them reach the egg. If an egg is fertilized, the coil stops the egg settling in the womb lining.

Advantages
➤ Provide very effective, long-term contraception. Failure rates for all copper coils are 1–2 percent.
➤ A coil can stay in place, and work, for a minimum of five years. Some coils, such as the Multi-load 375 and Ortho Gyne-T 380, are effective for seven years.

➤ They are effective as soon as they are put in, and can be used as an emergency contraceptive.

➤ It's a method that's easily reversible. The device is simply removed, and normal fertility returns immediately.

➤ Allows spontaneous sex, with no mess.

Disadvantages

➤ Periods can be heavier, more prolonged, and more painful.

➤ There may be spotting in-between periods.

➤ IUDs can increase the risk of a sexually transmitted infection spreading from the vagina to the womb and Fallopian tubes. This can lead to a severe pelvic infection, with subsequent scarring and fertility problems.

➤ Insertion of the device can be painful (especially in women who have never been pregnant) and can cause cramps afterwards.

➤ The womb can be damaged during insertion of the device. Occasionally, the wall of the womb is perforated, and the device placed outside the womb, in the pelvic cavity.

➤ Occasionally, the strings get caught up around the device, and are not visible through the cervix. This can make removal difficult.

➤ If you fall pregnant with a coil in place, there's an increased risk of the pregnancy being in the Fallopian tube (an ectopic). If the pregnancy is in the womb, there's an increased risk of mis-carriage, together with an infection afterwards. Anyone who suspects they are pregnant with a coil in place should see their doctor as soon as possible.

Because of the risks of severe infections, coils are not really suitable for women who have multiple sexual partners, or for those who have never been pregnant. Women who have never been pregnant also tend to suffer more from bleeding and pain after insertion. The coil should also be avoided by women who have had an ectopic preg-nancy in the past. They are most suitable for women who are either in-between babies, or whose families are complete (but who do not want to take a final, irreversible step).

All women should have a thorough check-up before a coil is inserted, to exclude any infection, such as chlamydia, that could be aggravated by a coil. Coils should also always be inserted by doctors thoroughly trained, and familiar with the technique.

BARRIER METHODS

These include condoms (for men and women), caps and diaphragms, and the sponge.

In general, barrier methods aren't as reliable as contraceptives when compared to hormonal methods, and so are not suitable for women whose number one requirement is protection from an unwanted pregnancy. However, barrier methods are becoming increasingly popular because they offer far better protection than other methods against sexually transmitted diseases, including HIV.

If you are in a new relationship you should use a barrier method for this reason, even if you are on the Pill. There's no harm in having the best of both worlds!

F

Male condom
This is still by far the most popular contraceptive method in use today in this country. The thin rubber sheath should be rolled carefully over the erect penis, after the air has been gently squeezed out the tip. Condoms work by preventing sperm from entering the vagina.

Advantages
➤ Easy to obtain direct from chemists – though if you go to a Family Planning clinic you can get them free.
➤ Fairly reliable if used correctly.
➤ Quick and easy to use.
➤ If used properly, offers excellent protection against sexually transmitted diseases, including AIDS, and can also help to prevent cancer of the cervix.
➤ No mess, and no smell, as the man's ejaculate is contained within the sheath.
➤ Makes the man take responsibility for contraception!

Disadvantages
➤ Not as reliable as some other methods. Failure rates vary enormously, and can be as high as 15 percent if they're not handled carefully.
➤ Putting it on can interrupt lovemaking
➤ If condoms are not put on correctly they may come off or split.
➤ Sheaths should always be put on before the penis touches a woman's vagina, as millions of sperm are present in the first few drops of semen that appear on the penis tip when it becomes erect.
➤ It's essential the man withdraws as soon as he has ejaculated, holding the sheath on to the penis so that no semen is accidently spilt.
➤ Both men and women can become allergic to sheath rubber, or lubricants. Special 'allergy' condoms can help to overcome this problem.

If you buy your own condoms, be sure to choose a brand marked with a BSI kitemark. Check the expiry date too! For extra protection, you can use sheaths together with vaginal spermicides (pessaries are particularly suitable). Avoid using any oil-based lubricants, such as body oils or Vaseline, as these can damage the rubber. If necessary, use a water-based lubricant, such as K-Y jelly, instead.

F

Female condom (The Femidom)
This is a soft polyurethane sheath, with a flexible supportive ring at each end, which is inserted into the vagina, and prevents sperm from entering the womb. A Femidom is much larger than an ordinary male sheath, and has been unfortunately likened to a plastic bag!

Advantages
➤ The failure rate of Femidoms has never been properly assessed in large-scale trials, but it's thought to be as reliable as the male condom – in other words, better than nothing at all, but not as good as many other methods.
➤ Easy to buy directly from chemists.
➤ Probably offers excellent protection against infections.
➤ Can be put in any time before sex.

Disadvantages
➤ Expensive and not easy to obtain free from GP's surgeries.
➤ Doesn't look very appealing, and the lubricant that covers the plastic can make it a bit slippery.

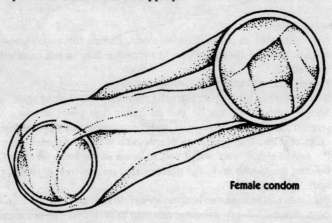

Female condom

➤ Some men have been known to miss the correct opening, and insert their penis between the Femidom and the vaginal wall.

Diaphragms and Caps

These are special rubber devices that are inserted into the vagina to cover the cervix and should be used together with a spermicide cream, or pessaries. They work by preventing sperm reaching the womb. If any sperm do leak out from around the edge of the device, they are killed by the action of the spermicide cream. Caps can be inserted up to two hours before sex, but must stay in place for at least six hours afterwards. Diaphragms, which are by far the most commonly used, are large devices that cover the whole of the front wall of the vagina as well as the cervix. Cervical caps are much smaller, and are attached, by suction, on to the cervix. Both come in a variety of sizes.

Advantages

➤ Fairly effective. Failure rates vary between 4–8 percent, depending largely on how carefully the device is used.
➤ With practise, many women find caps quick and easy to use, and because they can be put in up to two hours before sex, they don't have to interrupt lovemaking.
➤ Offer some protection against sexually transmitted infections and cervical cancer.

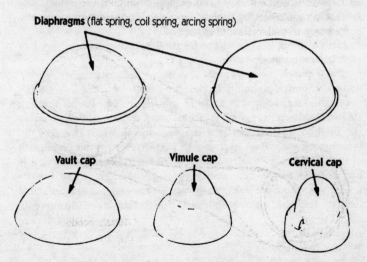

Diaphragms (flat spring, coil spring, arcing spring)

Vault cap　　　**Vimule cap**　　　**Cervical cap**

Disadvantages
➤ Not as effective as many other methods. Must be the correct size, which means a special fitting by a doctor or nurse is required.
➤ Can be fiddly, difficult and messy to use at first.
➤ Unless it's already in place, can interrupt lovemaking (inserting a cap can be more disruptive than slipping on a condom).
➤ Recurrent cystitis can be a problem for some diaphragm users. Switching to a type with a softer, more flexible rim, or a cervical cap, often solves this problem.
➤ If you have sex more than once, extra spermicide is required.
Caps should be checked regularly for holes, or shape distortion. They should be replaced at least once a year, and the size checked after having a baby or a miscarriage, or if you lose or gain more than 3kg. Caps are suitable for women who do not wish to use hormones, but they need to be used with great care to avoid an unwanted pregnancy.

Natural methods
These rely on body signals and menstrual patterns to tell you when you are at the most fertile time of the month. From this, it's possible to work out when it's safe to have unprotected intercourse, on the basis that sperm can live in a woman's body for up to five days, but the egg only survives for twenty-four hours after ovulation. There are only a few days in every cycle that you are actually fertile.

The method involves taking your temperature at the beginning of each day, (there's a rise just before ovulation), together with detecting changes in the cervical mucus (it becomes more runny and abundant around the time of ovulation).

Natural methods can either be used on their own, or together with barrier methods on 'unsafe days'.

The 'Persona' contraceptive system is a more scientific 'natural' method of family planning. By detecting changes in the levels of the two hormones, oestrogen and LH (see page 119), in the urine, a simple colour-coded system indicates 'safe' and 'unsafe' days. Using the method involves doing a simple urine test first thing in the morning for eight days each month (sixteen days in the first month of use). Used correctly, the system is 93–5 percent reliable, but it is not suitable for women with very erratic periods, those breast-feeding or who have polycystic ovaries. One major disadvantage is its cost – the basic kit costs £50, and urine test strips are £10 a month.

Advantages
➤ No side-effects.

➤ No 'interference' with natural body functions.
➤ No mess.
➤ Completely natural lovemaking on 'safe' days.
➤ The use of barrier methods only on fertile days.
➤ Increased self-awareness.
➤ Acceptable to some religious organisations that otherwise don't approve of contraception.

Disadvantages
➤ Can be very unreliable. Failure rates vary between 2–20 percent.
➤ Needs expert teaching from a nurse or doctor specially trained in the method.
➤ Involves the commitment of keeping daily records of body symptoms.
➤ Women with erratic periods, especially after childbirth or around the menopause, may find the method very difficult (though not impossible).

STERILIZATION
This is a surprisingly popular option – one in three couples around the world opt for it. Although in some cases it is possible to reverse a sterilization procedure, it must be regarded as a permanent form of contraception. Both men and women can be sterilised. The operation is much quicker and easier on the man, where it can be performed under a local anaesthetic. In women, a general anaesthetic is required. Anyone considering sterilization should have full counselling. It's not a decision anyone should make overnight – think about it very carefully. If you have any doubts at all, no matter how small, then abandon the idea!

You do not need to get your partner's consent to be sterilized, although obviously it's better if you do.

Female sterilization
This is done by blocking the fallopian tubes by either clips, rings, or heat diathermy (using electric heat to destroy the tissue). Occasionally the tubes are cut and tied. This means that the egg and sperm cannot meet. The operation is done via a laparoscope (see page 118), and involves a general anaesthetic. In nearly all cases, it's done on a day-case basis – an overnight stay in hospital isn't necessary.

Advantages
➤ It is very effective (though very occasionally pregnancies do occur afterwards – it is NOT 100 percent safe).

➤ It's permanent. You don't have to worry about contraception ever again!
➤ It is effective immediately after the operation.

Disadvantages
➤ It involves having a minor operation, with a general anaesthetic.
➤ It can cause abdominal discomfort for at least a week afterwards.
➤ Occasionally the operation fails, and if so, there's an increased chance of an ectopic pregnancy.
➤ You can't change your mind afterwards. Pregnancy rates after reversal procedures are exceedingly low.
➤ Occasionally, periods are slightly heavier after the operation. This is thought to be because of changes to the blood supply to the womb.

Male sterilization (a vasectomy)
This involves cutting and tying the tubes that lead from the testes to the penis. It's done via a tiny cut on each side of the groin, beside the top of the scrotum.

Sperm only make up a tiny part of ejaculate, which looks the same afterwards – most of it is glandular secretions.

Advantages
➤ Permanent, effective, contraception, though like female sterilisation, it's not foolproof. The failure rate is about 0.1 percent.
➤ It's quick and easy (usually taking about fifteen minutes) and can be done under local anaesthetic.

Disadvantages
➤ It can take three to six months for all the sperm to disappear from the ejaculate. Additional precautions are needed until two tests have confirmed that there are no sperm.
➤ Occasionally there may be problem at the operation site afterwards, such as bruising or an infection.
➤ Reversal procedures have a very low success rate.
➤ Don't be misled by a new partner who says he's had a vasectomy (an old ploy when he has no condoms). Check for the tiny scars!

FIBROMYALGIA
Also known as fibrositis, this is a condition that causes aching, stiff muscles, particularly in the lower back, neck, shoulders and thighs. Sufferers also tend to have several very tender points, often in the

neck, knee, shoulders, on the inside of the elbow and on the outside of the hip joint. It's a condition that's especially common in middle-aged women, who often have other, more general symptoms, such as tiredness, anxiety, headaches and irritable bowel syndrome (IBS). The cause isn't known, but it is often stress related. Keeping active is a vital part of treatment, and regular, gentle exercise can ease pain and stiffness. Some patients are also helped by anti-depressant drugs, together with anti-inflammatory painkillers.

F

FOOT PROBLEMS

Considering that feet carry the weight of the body, and walk an average 100,000 miles in a lifetime, they are often a very neglected part of a woman's body. The heavy wear and abuse that they are often subjected to means that foot problems are exceedingly common.

CORNS

These are thickened areas or plugs of skin found on the top and at the base of the toes and on the soles of the feet. They're caused by chronic pressure, usually from tight shoes. Wearing a corn pad and roomy shoes can ease discomfort, and the corn itself can usually be filed or cut away by a chiropodist.

ATHLETES FOOT

This is a fungal infection, which causes moist, itchy, flaking skin, usually between the toes. It can be effectively treated with anti-fungal cream or powder, or by using tea-tree oil, available directly from chemists. It can usually be prevented by wearing cotton tights or socks wherever possible, and by wearing leather not synthetic shoes (this includes the lining as well). Furry slippers should be avoided too! Better still is to go barefoot whenever you can. This helps to prevent excess sweat collecting between toes. Persistent athletes foot can be treated with new, more powerful anti-fungal creams and tablets, available on prescription from your GP.

VERUCCAS

These are ingrowing warts, found on the soles of the feet, and the toes. They're caused by a viral infection, usually picked up from a changing-room floor. Small ones often disappear of their own accord, though this may take several months. Larger, painful verrucas that are spreading, can either be treated by salicylic acid paint (available from chemists) together with regular filing, or with a blast of liquid nitrogen – available either at your GP's surgery, a chiropodist, or from your local hospital dermatology department.

INGROWING TOE NAILS
These are shiny, red, swollen and painful areas at the side of a nail, usually on the big toe. They're caused by a splinter of nail growing and digging into the flesh, almost always because the nail has been cut too curved down the side. They often become infected. Though some ingrowing toe nails do eventually settle of their own accord as the nail grows out, they often require surgical treatment in which a wedge has to be removed from the offending nail.

BUNIONS
These are prominent, lumpy, and sometimes tender joints, at the base of the big toe. They tend to run in families, but wearing tight-fitting, pointed shoes always makes them worse. Large bunions can be treated by corrective surgery to straighten and seal the deformed joint.

CHILBLAINS
These are itchy, purply red swellings that appear on the toes in cold weather. They're caused by narrowing of the blood vessels in the feet, and tight footwear always makes them worse. Applying talc may help to relieve the itching, but more important still is to keep feet warm at all times and to improve circulation in general by taking exercise and stopping smoking.

Self-help and prevention
Nearly all foot problems can easily be prevented by treating your feet with just a little more respect!
➤ The right footwear is essential. There should be enough room for your toes to wriggle slightly – they shouldn't rub against the sides. Pointed shoes should be reserved for special occasions only!
➤ Very high-heeled shoes push your foot forwards, and crush the toes against the front of your shoes. Keep heels low for everyday use.
➤ Cut your nails straight across. Don't curve the scissors down at the sides, and don't go digging underneath the nail corners with scissors either!
➤ Warm, sweaty feet are an ideal breeding ground for fungi and bacteria. Wash your feet every day with mild soap and water, drying carefully afterwards between your toes. Change your tights or socks every day as well.
➤ Wear proper, supportive trainers for exercise.

G

GALLSTONES

Gallstones are surprisingly common, especially in older women who are overweight. In many people gallstones don't cause any symptoms at all, and remain undetected until spotted on an X-ray!

The gallbladder is a small, pear-shaped sac under the liver, in the top right-hand side of the abdominal cavity. It stores bile which is produced in the liver, to aid the digestion of fats. Gallstones form when there's an abnormality in bile – usually because there's too much cholesterol present. The stones rub against the lining of the gallbladder, causing inflammation. The main symptom they cause is pain, which can be severe, particularly after a fatty meal (when the gall bladder empties), together with nausea and vomiting.

Occasionally gallstones pass into, and block, the bile duct – the tiny tube that takes bile into the intestine. As well as causing agonizing pain, this condition can also lead to jaundice.

Though gallstones can often be spotted on an ordinary X-ray, they are best diagnosed by an ultrasound scan.

Occasionally a long course of special tablets will successfully dissolve the stones. But in many cases the best treatment is to surgically remove the gallbladder. This is increasingly done laparoscopically (the key hole method) rather than through a large cut. Treatment is only needed if gallstones are causing a lot of symptoms. Occasional abdominal pain can often be kept at bay by avoiding fatty meals. Women with gallstones should also avoid using the combined contraceptive pill.

GARDNERELLA VAGINALIS

Gardnerella is bacteria that are normally found in very small numbers in the vagina. Any increase in their numbers can lead to creamy discharge, which usually has a noticeable fishy smell. The vagina may also feel sore (but not usually itchy). Though gardnerella may be sexually transmitted, in many women the infection occurs because of a change in the natural vaginal environment. This can be due to overwashing or douching (which washes away the vagina's natural protective secretions) or a hormonal change, such as starting the pill, or at the menopause.

The fishy smell is a very good diagnostic clue, which can be confirmed by a swab test done by your GP. Treatment is with the antibiotic metronidazole.

GONORRHOEA

This is the second most common sexually transmitted infection in the UK (NSU is the most common, see page 41). It's caused by the bacterium Neisseria Gonorrhoea. It's important that it is detected early especially in women as the infection can spread from the vagina and cervix up into the womb and Fallopian tubes, causing pelvic inflammatory disease (PID), and often subsequent infertility.

In men, gonorrhoea often produces a very noticeable thick, greeny discharge from the penis, but in women the picture is very different. There may be a slight creamy discharge, and infection around the urethra can cause a burning sensation when passing urine. These symptoms usually begin within two to ten days of contact with the infection, but in over half of women with the infection there are no symptoms at all till the pain of PID begins.

Gonorrhoea can be transmitted during oral sex, causing a sore throat, and a mother can also pass it on to her baby during childbirth, infecting the eyes, and causing conjunctivitis. Gonorrhoea can also occasionally spread into the blood stream through the womb lining, causing fever and joint pains.

Gonorrhoea can be effectively treated with antibiotics, but special high doses may be required. Even if you have no symptoms, if you suspect you may have had contact with gonorrhoea it's advisable to go to your local hospital department of genito-urinary medicine for tests. Just one cautionary check-up could protect your fertility for the future!

H

HAIR PROBLEMS

The only parts of the body which are completely hairless are the soles of the feet and the palms of the hands. The majority of the rest of the body is covered in fine hairs that are barely noticeable unless you're shivering, when they stand up. Thicker, coloured hairs normally only grow on the scalp, across the eyebrows, in the pubic area, and in the armpits.

EXCESS HAIR

At least 10 percent of women suffer from excess body hair. Thicker, coloured hair, like that in the armpits, can be found anywhere on the body, but the most common sites are the face, especially across the upper lip; the lower legs; the arms; and an extension of the pubic hair which grows up the tummy; and down the thighs.

Many darker-skinned women naturally inherit a tendency toward excess hair, and although this can be a cosmetic problem, it's not a health problem. However, in other women, excess hair can be an indication of an underlying hormonal imbalance. It's normal for all women to have small amounts of the male hormone testosterone, but women with excess hair often have excessive amounts. To make matters worse, this can lead to thinning of scalp hair, just like the early stages of baldness in men. This may be an isolated problem, or there may be an associated imbalance of the hormones that control menstruation; or be a symptom of tiny cysts in the ovaries – a condition known as PCO (see page 144).

As well as excess body hair, PCO sufferers often have a greasy skin and acne (due to high testosterone levels) and erratic periods.

In older, post-menopausal women, a slightly different hormone imbalance, mainly linked to low levels of oestrogen, can lead to more obvious facial hair growth.

Excess body hair can also be due to drugs, in particular phenytoin (used to treat epilepsy), danazol (used to treat endometriosis) and high doses of steroids. Female athletes who abuse anabolic steroids to increase their performance can have a severe problem with hairiness and have to shave each day.

Self-help for excess hair
There are several different ways of removing excess hair. None of them will stimulate hair growth, or make a hair problem worse – it may only feel this way because the short ends of regrowth are more bristly than longer hairs.

➤ The easiest way to get rid of excess hair is by shaving, although it's difficult to get a very smooth skin this way.

➤ Depilatory creams dissolve the hair above the skin and usually give a better cosmetic result than shaving. However, they can cause soreness and irritation, especially on women with sensitive skins.

➤ Waxing and sugaring pull out hairs from the root, and there may not be any really noticeable regrowth for several weeks afterwards.

➤ The only way to get a permanent cure is by electrolysis. A tiny electrical current is passed through the hair follicle, destroying the root. Unfortunately, it has several drawbacks. It's not available on the NHS, and as only a few follicles can be treated at each session, it can be a time-consuming and very expensive method of treatment. Treating a large area can also be quite painful. It's also very important that electrolysis is done by a person who is fully trained and qualified in the technique.

If you have a lot of excess hair, or if you suffer from erratic periods or a greasy skin, you should see a doctor.

Help from your doctor
➤ Hormone blood tests can confirm an excess of testosterone. This can be treated using the androgen blocker, cyproterone acetate, either on its own, or more commonly together with a low dose of oestrogen in the form of the contraceptive pill Dianette.

➤ A referral to a consultant dermatologist can be arranged for severe cases.

➤ Hormone-replacement therapy (HRT) can sometimes reduce excess hair in older women.

➤ Local anaesthetic creams are available on prescription that can ease the pain of electrolysis.

THINNING HAIR
The constant turnaround of new hairs replacing old ones means it's normal to lose up to 100 hairs from the scalp each day. For people with long hair, this can look quite a large amount. Some women have naturally thinner hair than others, but any sudden change, with the appearance of very thin, or even bald patches, needs investigating.

There are two main types of hair loss in women.

❶ Completely bald patches, with otherwise perfectly normal hair, are usually due to a condition known alopecia areata. This can be either due to a thyroid disorder, or the body's own immune system reacting against the hair follicles. However, often the cause isn't clear, but it can be stress related. Usually just a small area of scalp is affected, but very occasionally hair is lost from the whole of the head, and eyebrows and eyelashes fall out too.

❷ The second type, where the hair becomes generally thinner, is much more common. This can be due to:

➤ having a baby! It's common for there to be marked hair loss starting about three months after the birth, and continuing until the baby is about a year old. Changing hormone levels are to blame
➤ severe emotional stress, such as a bereavement or divorce
➤ severe illness, or crash dieting
➤ severe iron or zinc deficiency
➤ excess levels of the male hormone testosterone, which causes thinning on the top and side of the head ('male pattern' baldness)
➤ low levels of oestrogen after the menopause
➤ some cancer treatments.

Self-help for thinning hair
➤ Your hair needs proper nourishment to grow properly. Eat a well-balanced, nutritious diet, with red meat and green vegetables (to provide iron), seafood, dairy products and pumpkin seeds (to provide zinc).
➤ Try and reduce your stress levels (see page 161) – a vitamin B supplement may help if hair loss is stress related.
➤ Treat your hair gently. Avoid harsh chemical treatments, especially perms or strong bleaching, if possible. Use a wide-toothed comb or vent brush for styling. Avoid tightly packed bristle brushes that are more likely to tear your hair. Avoid tangles by using a good conditioner. If you style by blow-drying, use the low heat setting and keep the dryer at least six inches from your hair.
➤ Minoxidil lotion, now available from chemists, can help to promote hair growth, but this should only be used with the recommendation of a doctor.

Help from your doctor
➤ A blood test can confirm either iron or zinc deficiency. In these cases, a daily supplement may be useful.

➤ An underactive thyroid gland, leading to thyroid deficiency, can also be detected via a blood test. Treatment is with thyroid hormone tablets.

➤ Excessive testosterone can also be diagnosed via a blood test. Treatment is usually with the anti-androgen, cyproterone acetate.

➤ Hormone-replacement therapy (HRT) can help to stop hair loss in post-menopausal women.

➤ In severe cases, your GP can arrange a referral to a dermatologist.

HEADACHES

Headaches are the most common health problem in women. It's extremely rare to find someone who has never had one! They are particularly common in women during the reproductive years, and at least 75 percent of women have a headache of some sort at least once a month.

Headaches vary enormously in their severity, from a dull ache behind the eyes, or a slight heavy-headed feeling, to a severe pain that stops normal activities.

Most headaches are caused by tension and stress. But they can also be caused by changes in the blood vessels inside the head, toothache, sinusitis, and food intolerance. They can also be caused by sudden caffeine withdrawal, hunger or dehydration, particularly when it's caused by an excess of alcohol! They can also be caused by some medications) particularly in women by hormonal contra-ceptives), and occasionally hormone-replacement therapy (HRT). Any acute illness, particularly one that causes a fever, can cause a headache. But a headache on it's own is very rarely the sign of any serious illness.

Tension headaches are commonly caused by tiredness, stress or anxiety. The pain typically occurs either behind the eyes, across the forehead, or across the top of the head. Tension headaches are often linked with a slightly stiff, tender neck – which on its own can be a sign of anxiety and stress. Tension headaches can become a chronic problem that occurs on waking and lasts right through the day with increasing severity.

A sinus headache is usually a throbbing pain, which can be quite severe, across the top of the eyes, and across the cheeks, that's worse on bending down.

A headache that starts behind the eyes, and then extends into the head can also be a sign of eye strain, and a need for corrective glasses.

Self-help for headaches
➤ Take a painkiller, such as paracetamol, aspirin, or ibuprofen.
➤ Try and relax – the best way is to have a short rest with your eyes closed. If you're at work, take a break from your VDU screen.
➤ Have a long relaxing bath with a few drops of lavender oil added. If you're tense, ask a friend to give your shoulders and neck a gentle massage.
➤ A gentle massage of the temples can also be soothing.
➤ Headache related to blocked sinuses can often be relieved by a steam inhalation, with a few drops of menthol and eucalyptus oil added to the water.
➤ If you're having frequent headaches, have an eye test to check if you need glasses.

H

Help from your doctor
Though headaches are rarely due to a serious health problem, any woman having recurrent headaches (more than three regularly each month), or a sudden severe headache, should see their doctor. The examination should include a blood pressure check. You should also discuss whether any medications you are taking, particularly hormones, could be to blame, and consider a change of formulation.

Prevention
➤ Eat regular meals. Hunger and a low blood sugar are a common cause of headache.
➤ Cut down on your alcohol (particularly red wine) and caffeine intake.
➤ Avoid getting overtired.
➤ Reduce your stress levels as much as you can (see page 161).
➤ Make sure your workplace is well ventilated.
➤ Check your diet, and eliminate any foods that may be causing headaches. Excessive amounts of synthetic colourings and flavourings, particularly monosodium glutamate, are often to blame.

MIGRAINE
This is a specific type of headache, caused by changes in the blood vessels inside the brain. These changes are thought to be caused by tiny changes in the level of the brain chemical, serotonin. The result is a severe, thumping headache pain that can last anything from two hours to two days. Only one side of the head is usually affected. The headache is usually preceded by flashing lights in the eyes, and nausea or vomiting.

Migraines can also cause symptoms elsewhere in the body, particularly pins and needles, or numbness, and occasionally weakness in one hand, which spreads up the arm to involve the face.

Women are affected by migraine three times more commonly than men, mainly because they can be triggered by the changing hormone levels that occur as part of the menstrual cycle. Migraines can occur at any age, but they usually start before the age of thirty. Migraines suddenly occurring in an older person should always be promptly investigated by a doctor.

Migraine attacks often start for no reason, but can be triggered by stress, anxiety, a change of routine, or even a change of climate. Some foods, especially chocolate, cheese, red wine and citrus fruits (especially oranges), may also be to blame.

H

Self-help
➤ Keep a food diary to try and identify, and then avoid, any possible food triggers for attacks.
➤ Take action as soon as you get the first symptoms of an attack. Don't wait until the pain is severe. Get home as soon as possible, and lie down in a dark room. Don't be tempted to relax in front of the TV – the flickering screen can make a migraine worse.
➤ Simple painkillers, such as aspirin and paracetamol often only just take the edge off migraine pain. Try a more powerful painkiller containing a combination of paracetamol with either codeine, or stronger still, dihydrocodeine. High dose ibuprofen (400mg, every eight hours) may also help. If nausea is a problem, try Migraleve, which contains an anti-sickness ingredient in addition to strong painkillers.
➤ Feverfew is a natural remedy that can reduce the frequency and severity of migraine attacks. For good effect you need to take a daily tablet for at least two months. Choose a formulation containing at least 0.2 percent of the active ingredient parthenolide for every 125mg of feverfew leaf powder.

Help from your doctor.
➤ Menstrual migraine, which occurs around the time of a period, can often be relieved by hormone treatment. However, the combined pill can make migraines worse, and should definitely be avoided if you suffer from weakness or tingling, or severe eye symptoms as part of a migraine attack.
➤ Stronger painkillers and anti-sickness drugs are available on prescription.

➤ Drugs that can reduce the severity of migraine attacks include ergotamine, and better still, sumatriptan. For best effect, both should be used as soon as symptoms of a migraine start.

➤ For frequent migraine attacks (more than once a month), it's worthwhile considering preventative treatment. These need to be taken all the time, and not just during an attack. Drugs available for this purpose include beta-blockers and pizotifen.

HEART

Many women mistakenly believe that cancer is the biggest threat to their health. They're wrong. In this country, it's heart disease that's the biggest health threat, for women as well as men – a quarter of all women die from it. Every year, five times more women die from coronary heart disease than from breast cancer.

Most heart disease is caused by thickening of the lining of the arteries that supply the heart – atherosclerosis. This reduces the blood and oxygen supply to the heart muscle, making it weaker. If one of the arteries blocks completely, this prevents any oxygen reaching a portion of the muscle – a heart attack.

For many women, the first sign that they have heart disease is the sudden, excruciating pain of a heart attack. Others suffer for years from breathlessness and chest pain (angina) on even slight exertion, which can ruin their quality of life. Worse still, many women feel constantly on edge, and unable to relax, as they never know when a fatal attack is going to strike.

Heart disease doesn't just affect older women. Increasing numbers of younger women – some still in their thirties – are suffering from angina and even heart attacks. Anyone can be affected, but some are more at risk than others. This includes:

➤ smokers. Smoking more than doubles the chance of a heart attack, and for those under fifty, smokers are five times more likely to die of heart disease compared to non-smokers

➤ those with high blood pressure. This puts an increased strain on the heart. The higher the pressure, and the longer it goes untreated, the greater the risk

➤ those with a family history of heart disease. Even if you are otherwise completely healthy, if heart disease runs in your family you're at increased risk of suffering from it too

➤ those who are overweight. Obesity by itself puts an increased strain on the heart, and also increases the risk of diabetes and high blood pressure. Women who are 'apple' shaped, with most of their excess weight around their waists, are more at risk of heart disease than those who are 'pear' shaped, with excess fat around their hips

➤ those with a high blood cholesterol level. Too much cholesterol, especially the high density lipoprotein fraction (HDL) can accelerate the formation of atherosclerosis.

Self help

With heart disease, prevention is all important. You can help to keep your heart healthy by making a few lifestyle adjustments. The earlier you take action, the better your chances of living a long and healthy life – but it's never too late to start! You should:

➤ take regular exercise. This boosts the circulation, and helps to keep the heart muscle in good condition. You don't need to 'go for the burn' – twenty minutes of gentle exercise that makes you slightly puffed is good enough – but you should aim to do this at least three times a week

➤ stop smoking

➤ if you are overweight go on a sensible diet

➤ take hormone-replacement therapy (HRT) after the menopause (see page 96)

➤ adjust your diet by:

   ➤ cutting down on fatty foods, especially those containing animal fats, such as butter, cream, sausages and meat pies

   ➤ throwing away the frying pan. Grill or bake foods instead

   ➤ eating more fresh fruit and vegetables, especially citrus fruit, carrots and green leafy vegetables, which are good sources of the anti-oxidants beta carotene and vitamins C and E, which can help prevent heart disease

   ➤ eating more oily fish, such as salmon and herring. Their oils, known as Omega 3 fish oils, are now known to help prevent heart disease

   ➤ using oat-based cereals where possible. Oats have been shown to help reduce cholesterol levels

   ➤ cutting down on salt and salty foods. Too much salt can increase blood pressure

   ➤ eating garlic on a regular basis – it's been shown to have a beneficial effect on the heart

   ➤ drinking alcohol in moderation. Rather surprisingly, several research studies have shown that regular small amounts of alcohol can help prevent heart disease. It's still unclear whether wine is best, or whether alcohol in any form, such as

H

spirits, will do! But don't drink more than fourteen units a week, or you'll risk other health problems (see page 12).

Supplements
There is some evidence that even if you have a good diet, taking certain supplements may help prevent heart disease. They include:
➤ Vitamins A, C and E, and beta carotene. These are called anti-oxidants because they mop up molecules known as free radicals, that can damage healthy cells
➤ omega 3 fish oils. The most well-known of these is cod liver oil
➤ garlic. Capsules are available which don't make your breath smell!

Help from your doctor
Even if you feel perfectly well, it is worthwhile seeing your doctor once every three years for a check on your blood pressure, and cholesterol level. This applies particularly to those in the high risk groups.

H

HERPES
This is an infection caused by the Herpes Simplex group of viruses. Any part of the body can be affected, but the two most common sites are around the lips (often known as cold sores), and around the genital area.

The first symptom is usually tingling of the affected skin, which is followed in the next twenty-four hours by a collection of blisters. These break down, again usually within a day, to form acutely painful ulcers. These gradually scab over, usually within a week.

Herpes is passed on by direct contact with the open sores. The incubation period is usually just a few days, but can be up to a week. People with cold sores should take care to avoid kissing anyone else, and those with genital sores should avoid close sexual contact. Once the skin has healed over it's perfectly safe to resume normal activities. If you are pregnant then your midwife and/or doctor should be informed that you have the virus as there is a slight chance that the baby can be infected during labour if active spots are present.

Recurrences – the facts
Herpes has been the subject of many scary stories because the virus can lay dormant inside the body in nerve cells, and then suddenly become active again, causing recurrent attacks. At least 20 percent of people only ever have one herpes attack. Others only have

occasional recurrences, less than once a year. If recurrences do occur, they are rarely as painful as the first attack, heal up much quicker and tend to become less frequent with passing time, until they disappear altogether. More frequent attacks are often sparked off by a factor that can be identified, such as stress, cold or hot weather, sunlight, or hormonal changes at period times.

Self-help
Acyclovir (or Zovirax) is a powerful anti-viral drug that can reduce the severity of herpes attacks, making the ulcers less painful and speeding up the healing process. It works best if it's applied as soon as an attack starts. All herpes sufferers should keep a tube handy.

Passing urine can be agony during an attack of genital herpes. Drink plenty of fluids to dilute urine acid levels, and if necessary, pass urine in the bath.

H

Help from your doctor
Acyclovir tablets are more effective than the cream, but they are only available on prescription. If they're used at the start of an initial attack, they may prevent recurrences altogether. So see your doctor as soon as possible if you suspect you have genital herpes.

A long course of acyclovir tablets, taken for up to three months, may also help to stop frequent recurrent attacks.

HORMONE-REPLACEMENT THERAPY (HRT)
As its name suggests, HRT is a drug treatment which replaces the hormone oestrogen when it is no longer being produced naturally by the body. However, it's not suitable for women who've had womb cancer, and it should only be prescribed by experts for women who've had breast cancer. Women with a strong family history of breast cancer should also have expert advice before starting HRT.

In younger women, oestrogen is produced by the ovaries. Not only is oestrogen a vital part of the monthly menstrual cycle, but it also plays a very important part in keeping the heart and blood vessels healthy, and the bones strong. At the menopause, or if the ovaries are removed, oestrogen levels fall dramatically – causing, amongst other symptoms, the hot flushes and sweats that many women suffer from at this time. In the long term, low oestrogen levels allow heart disease and osteoporosis to develop at a rapid rate.

One of the other functions of oestrogen is to create a build-up in the lining of the womb. Before the menopause, this has the useful biological function of preparing the womb for a fertilized egg. If there's no pregnancy, the womb lining is shed naturally once a month, as a period. After the menopause, long-term oestrogen administration can lead to a very thick womb lining, erratic bleeding, and very occasionally, the development of abnormal cells, that can become cancerous. To counteract this, and to ensure that the womb lining stays thin and safe, all women on HRT must take a second hormone, progesterone, for some of the time. The most common regime is to give some sort of progesterone for twelve days each month, which will then induce a monthly bleed. However, new regimes are available now which mean that it's possible to have safe HRT without regular monthly periods (see below). Women who've had a hysterectomy don't need to bother about progesterone – all that's needed is oestrogen.

Advantages
There are plenty of very positive reasons for taking HRT. They include:
➤ it can relieve unpleasant menopausal symptoms such as hot flushes, sweats, tiredness, sleeping problems and depression
➤ it can relieve a dry, itchy vagina and make sex more comfortable
➤ it can help to keep the heart and circulation healthy, and so really can prolong life!
➤ it can help to prevent osteoporosis.

Disadvantages
As with so many good things in life, HRT has its fair share of disadvantages. These include:
➤ for many women (but not all) it means having periods again. However, these should be not be heavy
➤ some women find that HRT makes them feel a bit bloated, with tender breasts and a tendency to gain weight. These symptoms are more noticeable with higher dose formulations, and switching to a lower dose often helps
➤ the progesterone component can cause PMT-type symptoms, such as depression and mild acne
➤ there is some evidence that long-term use of HRT, for more than eight years, may increase the risk of developing breast cancer. However, more women die of heart disease than breast cancer, so this risk needs to be carefully weighed against the beneficial effects for the heart
➤ some HRT comes from horses' urine. This may affect your choice of pill.

Who, when and how long?

HRT is suitable for nearly all women. Unlike the combined contraceptive pill, which contains a relatively high dose of synthetic oestrogen, HRT contains a low dose of natural oestrogen, and this means it is suitable for many older women who were unable to take the Pill for medical reasons, such as a deep-vein thrombosis or high blood pressure. In fact, there are positive reasons for women with high blood pressure to take HRT!

It can be started as soon as there are symptoms of oestrogen deficiency, such as sweats – your periods do not have to have stopped. But if you are still having periods, it's a good idea to have a blood test first to check that you are approaching the menopause, and that your symptoms do not have another cause.

It's never to late to start HRT – women in their seventies can start treatment, and gain benefit. Ideally, to have a good effect on bones and the heart, treatment should continue for at least five years. Many women continue safely, and happily, much longer than this. But in the end it's a matter of individual choice. If you're not happy with it, or if you can't find a preparation that suits you, then you can stop treatment at any time (though it's best to complete a month's course, and have a withdrawal bleed).

Treatment choices

There's a bewildering array of different formulations of HRT available, and the choice is widening all the time. There are four main types of treatment – pills, patches, gel and implants. Oestrogen cream is also available for use in the vagina, to ease dryness.

With all the preparations, the higher the dose the greater the benefits will be, but also the greater the risk of unwanted side effects, such as heavy periods or weight problems.

Pills

Pills are the most popular choice. They come in a variety of different formulations, using different oestrogens and progesterones in varying strengths. In many cases, the progesterone component is combined with the oestrogen into a single pill. They are easy to take, and adjusting the dose is usually fairly straightforward.

Patches

Patches are worn on the skin below the waist. The hormone they contain is absorbed directly through the skin into the blood stream. This has the theoretical advantage of giving a constant blood level, and also of avoiding the liver – all oestrogen swallowed in pills has to pass through the liver before it reaches the blood stream.

Some women find that they suffer fewer side effects from patches compared to other methods. However, some women are allergic to them, and they do occasionally come off, especially in hot weather (there are reports of women waking in the morning to find their husband wearing the patch!). They should be worn all the time. The most common ones are changed twice weekly, though there are now new patches available that are changed only once a week.

The progesterone component can either be given in the form of a double patch, containing both hormones, or as separate pills.

Gel
Gel is a relatively new addition to the HRT range in this country, though it has been available (and very popular) in France for many years. Two pre-measured blobs of gel, containing oestrogen, are rubbed into the arms or thighs each day. It can be slightly messy and time-consuming to apply, but it does have the advantage of causing fewer allergic reactions than patches. For many women, the gel seems more like a beauty treatment than a medicine!

Implants
Impants are inserted under the skin of the abdomen under local anaesthetic. The oestrogen they contain is then slowly released into the blood stream for approximately the next six months. They are most suitable for women who have had a hysterectomy, although they can be used by others, as long as a regular monthly course of progesterone tablets is taken as well. Implants can give unpredictably high levels of oestrogen to some women.

Bleed-free HRT
This is now an option for many women who have not had a natural period for more than a year. One popular choice, Tibolone, is a completely new combination drug of oestrogen and progesterone. Occasional breakthrough bleeding may occur. The other choice, Kliofem, involves taking conventional oestrogen, but with continuous progesterone. It can cause erratic bleeding in the first few months of treatment. Another option is Tridestra, a special combination of hormones that induces a bleed once every three months. In the future, insertion of a Mirena coil may give many women on HRT very light, or virtually non-existent periods.

Don't be tempted to change your HRT too quickly. Give your body at least three months to get used to any preparation. But if it still doesn't suit you, don't be scared to go back to your doctor and ask to try something new. There are so many different choices available that eventually you should be able to find one that you like – but it can take a long time!

HYMEN

This is a thin membrane just inside the entrance to the vagina. It normally has a small central opening, which allows the flow of menstrual blood. This stretches using tampons, but on first intercourse the hymen usually tears, which may be slightly painful and can occasionally (but not always) cause slight bleeding.

Occasionally there is no central perforation, and menstrual blood collects in the vagina. This can easily be corrected by a simple operation.

HYSTEROSCOPY

This is an operation to examine the inside of the womb. It's done using a special fibre-optic telescope, which is passed into the womb through the vagina and cervix. It allows the surgeon to view any abnormality, such as a polyp, or fibroids, directly. It's increasingly used instead of a D and C (see page 51) as an investigation for abnormal bleeding. It's usually done under general anaesthetic, but an overnight stay in hospital isn't normally necessary.

HYSTERECTOMY

This is an operation to remove the womb. The womb may be removed on its own, or together with the Fallopian tubes and ovaries. It's a common operation in the UK – more than 1,000 women have it performed each week.

There are two main types of hysterectomy.

❶ An abdominal hysterectomy involves removing the womb through a cut in the lower tummy wall. This is usually done across the top of the pubic hairline, but occasionally, a vertical cut may be required straight down the middle of the lower tummy, below the tummy button.

❷ A vaginal hysterectomy involves removing the womb through a cut in the top of the vagina. The operation involves carefully

cutting and tying the blood vessels and ligaments to the womb –
it is NOT done by suction.

A vaginal hysterectomy has the advantage of not leaving any visible
scars, and recovery afterwards is often much quicker. However, it's
not suitable for all women as some wombs are too big to fit through
the vagina.

The womb only has two functions – it acts as an incubator for
babies during pregnancy, and it prepares the body to become pregnant on a monthly cycle – when pregnancy does not occur it sheds
its lining, usually once a month (a period). It does not produce any
hormones at all – they come from the ovaries. That means that
although removing the womb does mean no more periods, it doesn't
mean an instant menopause unless the ovaries are removed as well.
The continued cyclical secretion of hormones from the ovaries can
mean that some women who've had a hysterectomy continue to
suffer PMT-type symptoms each month – even though they don't
have periods!

Having a hysterectomy does mean saying a very final goodbye to
the chance of having any more children. To older women, who have
decided years before that their families were complete, this may not
be an issue. But it can be a major problem for younger women,
which is why any decision to have the operation should be considered very carefully, without rushing. It's not something that can be
put to rights later.

Reasons for having a hysterectomy include:
➤ heavy or painful periods (by far the most common reason)
➤ chronic pelvic inflammatory disease (PID), causing severe pain
➤ endometriosis
➤ lax womb ligaments leading to a prolapse – the most common
  reason for a vaginal hysterectomy
➤ large fibroids
➤ cancers of the cervix, womb or ovaries.

What's involved?
Having a hysterectomy no longer means a long hospital stay – many
women are discharged home three days afterwards. Women having
an abdominal hysterectomy may need fairly strong painkillers for a
week or so, but those having a vaginal operation may have remarkably little discomfort afterwards.

It takes at least six weeks, and often a lot longer, to make a full
recovery. Chronic tiredness, and a lack of energy are the most
common problems that women describe. All women should avoid

any heavy lifting for at least three months after the operation, but it's normally possible to resume a normal sex life after the routine six week check-up by your doctor.

Having a hysterectomy should not make you put on weight. The main reason that this occurs in some women is because they are very inactive afterwards, and indulge in too many chocolates! Women under forty-five who have their ovaries removed as well as the womb, should usually start HRT as soon as possible after the operation. This will prevent unpleasant menopausal symptoms, such as hot flushes, and also, more importantly, will help to prevent the early onset of osteoporosis and heart disease.

INCONTINENCE

Many women suffer needlessly from incontinence. There are two main types. They are treated differently, so it's important to work out which type is affecting you.

STRESS INCONTINENCE

This is accidently passing urine when extra pressure is put on the bladder, for example during running, coughing sneezing, or even just laughing. It's caused by weakness of the muscles around the base of the bladder and the pipe leading from the bladder, the urethra. It's a very common problem, especially when the pelvic floor muscles are stretched after childbirth.

Self-help for stress incontinence

Being overweight always makes incontinence worse – another good reason for really trying at that diet!

Stress incontinence can often be cured by toning and strengthening the pelvic-floor muscles. This is done by pelvic-floor exercises. To make any noticeable difference, you'll need to do the exercises several times a day for at least six months – so don't despair too soon!

❶ First of all, try stopping and starting the flow of urine when you go to the toilet. Do this until you feel you really have control of the flow – this will mean that you are good at tightening the muscles around your bladder.

❷ Next, exercise these muscles when you're not on the toilet. Sitting on a chair, squeeze hard, for a slow count of four, then relax.

❸ The next step is to work on the muscles further back, around your vagina and anus. Squeeze the muscles as if you were trying to stop yourself passing wind, or opening your bowels.

❹ Next, combine both exercises together. Again, hold for a slow count of four, then relax. Repeat at least five times.

Once you've mastered the pelvic-floor muscles, you can do these exercises at any time, such as doing the washing up, at work, or watching the T.V.. Aim to do them at least ten times each day.

If these exercises don't help (remember, you need to keep at them), then you may find using vaginal cones helpful. These are small plastic weights that look like tampons, which you hold in your vagina using your pelvic floor muscles. Alternatively, the muscles can be toned using a small electronic stimulator. These painless treatments are available via your local continence advisor. Ask your GP for a referral.

If these measures don't help, you may benefit from an operation to strengthen and support the base of the bladder. This can either be carried out through the vagina (a vaginal repair) or through the abdominal wall. It's important to have thorough investigations by a specialist first, including special X-rays of the bladder taken before and after you pass urine (a micturating cystogram). This can show whether surgery is likely to be helpful or not.

URGE INCONTINENCE

This is when there's a sudden uncontrollable urge to pass urine, at any time. 'Holding on' till you get to the toilet is nearly impossible. Once leaking starts, it can be difficult to control.

This type of incontinence may be due to a bladder infection, which can be cured by a short course of antibiotics from your GP. However, it's more commonly caused by irritable bladder muscles, which go into spasm for no obvious reason.

Self-help for urge incontinence
➤ Lose excess weight, which puts extra pressure on the bladder.
➤ Avoid caffeine, which can irritate the bladder.
➤ Don't drink excessive amounts of fluid – six to eight cups a day is enough unless the weather is very hot.
➤ Try to 'train' your bladder to hold more urine. Keep a record of how often you go and try and last at least two hours. While you're doing this, avoid going 'just in case'.

Urge incontinence can also be treated by special drugs that relax the bladder muscles, such as oxybutynin. Unfortunately, these often have side-effects, such as a dry mouth and constipation.

INFERTILITY

Infertility problems are surprisingly common. Figures vary, but between one in six to one in ten couples have difficulty in conceiving a child. The good news is that many of these do eventually, sooner or later, have a healthy baby.

Many couples start worrying far too soon that they have a fertility problem. Compared to animals, humans are very inefficient at reproduction. It's normal for it to take at least three months for a fertile woman in her twenties to conceive. A woman's fertility gradually declines from the early thirties onwards, and this figure rises to six months for a woman in her mid-thirties, even when there is absolutely nothing wrong. Even if a couple do have a problem, it's wrong to automatically assume the woman is to blame. It takes two to make a baby, and female fertility problems only account for 30 percent of cases. Male fertility problems account for another 30 percent, and in the remaining 40 percent, the reason for the problem is either a combination of both, or is never found (unexplained infertility).

Making babies – and why it goes wrong

To conceive, a sperm from the man needs to successfully fuse with an egg from the woman. The release of an egg from one of the ovaries (ovulation) usually occurs approximately mid-way between periods. When the egg is not fertilized, fourteen days usually pass between ovulation and the start of bleeding. This means that for a woman with a regular twenty-eight day cycle (that is, twenty-eight days between the start of one period and the next) ovulation occurs fourteen days after the start of a period. For a woman with a naturally longer cycle (say thirty-two days between periods) ovulation will occur four days later, around day eighteen. For shorter cycles (for instance twenty-five days between periods) ovulation will be around day eleven. The timing is important because the egg can only survive, and be fertilized, for twenty-four hours after it's released from the ovary. Sperm, on the other hand, can live for up to five days inside a woman's body.

This makes timing of intercourse important – but you don't need to make love every day. Once every two to three days is enough. But unless your partner has a low sperm count (see page 108), frequent intercourse, even several times a day, shouldn't do any harm! Aim for days nine to fourteen of your cycle.

For the sperm to meet the egg, they first have to penetrate through the mucus inside the cervix, then swim up through the womb, and Fallopian tubes. Any structural abnormality, or blockage in any part of the cervix, womb, and particularly the Fallopian tubes, can prevent the sperm from ever reaching the egg. For maximum fertility, ovulation needs to occur on a fairly regular basis, though many women with erratic cycles do manage to conceive without undue difficulty.

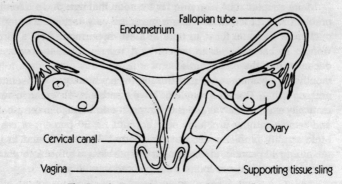

The Female Reproductive Tract (front view)

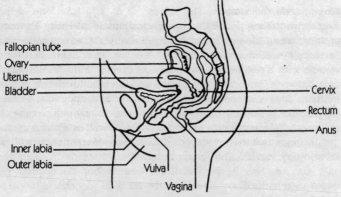

The Female Reproductive Tract (side view)

COMMON PROBLEMS IN WOMEN
Ovulation problems

These account for approximately one third of cases of female infertility. They can be caused by a hormone imbalance or by abnormalities in the ovaries themselves.

Ovulation is closely controlled by two hormones, FSH and LH (see page 119) produced by the pituitary gland in the brain. Any defect in their production (which normally varies at different times of the menstrual cycle) can lead to ovulation problems.

Excessive amounts of the hormone prolactin (also produced in the pituitary gland) and abnormalities in the amounts of thyroid hormone present, can also interrupt ovulation. High prolactin levels can be caused by a small tumour inside the pituitary gland.

Severe shock and stress can also affect hormone levels. Some doctors feel that the stress of worrying about getting pregnant is a cause of infertility in some women!

Often there's no underlying reason for hormone problems, but in an increasing number of women, low hormone levels are a result of an abnormally low body weight. Excessive amounts of exercise can also be to blame.

Polycystic ovaries, when tiny cysts form inside the ovarian tissue, is the most common ovarian cause of ovulation problems. Endometriosis inside the ovaries, surgical damage to the ovaries, and premature ovarian failure (when the ovaries don't respond to FSH and LH) are also, more rarely, to blame.

Blocked Fallopian tubes
This accounts for a further third of cases of female infertility. The most common reason is pelvic inflammatory disease (PID), when an infection first inflames, then scars and narrows, the delicate lining of either one, or both of the Fallopian tubes. The longer an infection goes untreated, the greater the chance of permanent damage. The tubes can also be damaged by an infection spreading from a burst appendix, or from endometriosis. Any infection, and also surgery to any of the organs in the lower abdomen (this includes the bowel as well as the ovaries and womb), can result in the formation of fine bands of scar tissue, or adhesions, which can distort or block the tubes.

Thickened cervical mucus
This accounts for approximately 5 percent of cases of female infertility. In some cases there is too little mucus present, but more common is mucus that is too thick for sperm to penetrate. Sometimes it also contains antibodies that destroy the sperm.

Problems in the womb
Problems such as large fibroids, or adhesions that cause the walls of the womb to stick together, or other abnormalities that are present from birth, can cause infertility. More commonly, however, these problems cause repeated early miscarriages.

COMMON PROBLEMS IN MEN
An amazingly large number of sperm are needed for normal fertility. Unlike the solitary egg, one sperm alone is not enough.

Before fertilization occurs, the egg is completely surrounded by sperm, which release chemicals that weaken the egg's tough outer covering. This allows a single sperm to penetrate inside the wall, and fertilize the egg.

It's not just numbers that count either. For good fertility, there must be a sufficient number of sperm of a normal shape and structure that can swim and progress up the woman's genital tract.

For fertility, an ejaculate of normal semen should:
➤ be more than 1.5ml in volume
➤ contain more than twenty million sperm in each ml
➤ have more than 70 percent of the sperm actively motile
➤ have more than 60 percent of the sperm structurally normal.

More than 90 percent of male infertility problems are because there are either too few sperm (and sometimes none at all), or because too many of them are structurally abnormal. This can be caused by:
➤ structural problems in the testis, such as undescended testes that are not lying in the scrotum, or a testes that has twisted in childhood and lost its blood supply (a torsion)
➤ hormonal problems
➤ enlarged veins around the testis (a varicocele), which causes overheating of the testis
➤ an infection in the testis, particularly mumps
➤ drugs, particularly anabolic steroids and marijuana.

Chemotherapy drugs used to treat cancer can also destroy the capacity of the testes to produce sperm. Excessive amounts of alcohol, nicotine and caffeine can also badly affect sperm production, but this is a reversible effect.

Sperm are produced best in a cool environment (which is why the testes lie outside the body). Any infection that causes a fever, such as a nasty bout of the 'flu, can cause a temporary fall in the sperm count. As sperm take three months to form, this will only be revealed in a semen analysis performed three months later. This also means it's always worth thinking back three months if the results of a semen analysis is poor. If so, repeat it again a month later to see if it's altered.

Self-help
Though infertility is often thought of as a problem that needs specialist and highly technical treatment, there is a lot you can do to maximize your chances of conceiving.
➤ Keep as healthy as possible by eating a well-balanced diet, taking a reasonable amount of exercise, and getting plenty of

sleep. All women trying for a baby should also take a daily supplement of 0.4mg folic acid, to help prevent spina bifida and brain defects in the baby.

➤ Stop smoking and cut your alcohol intake right down.

➤ Check your weight. If you are underweight it could stop regular ovulation, and there is also evidence that being very overweight can also affect fertility. Aim for a body mass index (see page 187) of between twenty and twenty-five.

➤ Don't let your life, and your relationship, become ruled by trying for a baby. There is some evidence that the stress of this alone can delay a pregnancy.

➤ Aim to have regular intercourse, at least once every two days, at your most fertile time. This is the week leading up to, and including, ovulation. But don't stop too soon, in case you ovulate later than normal.

Checking ovulation

You can check yourself when you ovulate by:

➤ taking your temperature each day. You need to do it first thing in the morning, before you get up, and before you have an early morning cup of tea or coffee. You need to use a special thermometer (available from chemists), and record the measurements on a chart. Your body temperature should rise by at least 0.4°C, and stay up, after ovulation. It falls again at the start of each period. Though temperature taking can be useful, especially if you're not sure when you ovulate, it can be unreliable (for instance, your temperature will go up if you have any type of infection, such as a nasty cold, or the 'flu). It also requires commitment, and can be a nasty daily reminder that you may have a fertility problem. Don't let your thermometer become an obsession – three months temperature taking is quite enough for anyone

➤ monitoring changes in your cervical and vaginal secretions. In the few days leading up to ovulation, they become much more plentiful, and are often apparent as a clear, vaginal discharge that may resemble egg white. This disappears the day after ovulation has occurred

➤ using an ovulation detector kit, also available from chemists. These use urine samples to detect the hormonal changes that occur at ovulation. Although they can be very accurate, they are also very expensive.

And for him

For a maximum sperm count, your partner should:

➤ stop smoking and drinking

➤ eat a healthy diet and take a reasonable amount of exercise

➤ avoid very long hot baths, and long sessions in steam rooms and saunas. Traditionally, men have also been advised to wear loose-fitting clothes (especially boxer shorts) and avoid tight underpants and jeans. However, for most men, the effect of tight clothing is probably negligible, and only becomes important when the sperm count is lower than normal.

Help from your doctor

Don't rush to your doctor's surgery too soon – give nature a chance! Women under thirty should usually actively 'try' for at least a year before seeking help, although women over thirty should seek help after six months. This is because fertility falls dramatically with increasing age (especially in women over thirty-five), and infertility tests and treatment can take months, and often years, to organize.

It's also worthwhile seeing your doctor a little sooner than normal if you, or your partner, have good reason to suspect that you have a problem that may mean you will need help to conceive. Indicators of this include

➤ very erratic periods, suggesting an ovulation problem.

➤ a previous confirmed diagnosis of polycystic ovaries, other hormone problems, or endometriosis

➤ severe pelvic inflammatory disease (PID) in the past

➤ an inflamed testis, or surgery to a testis in the past.

Try and see your doctor together, as a couple. Far too many women are left to carry the burden of the initial doctor's visit on their own. Going together will help both of you, and your doctor.

Tests

A good GP can arrange many of the initial tests, which will help to give an indication of where the problem may lie. These include:

➤ full hormone tests to check for ovulation. Two lots are usually required – one at the beginning of a period and another a week after presumed ovulation

➤ a semen analysis

➤ sometimes a pelvic ultrasound scan, if your doctor suspects you may have a structural abnormality, such as fibroids.

All women undergoing infertility tests should also make sure they are immune to rubella (this can be checked with a simple blood test), and also have had a cervical smear in the last three years. An HIV test is not usually done as a routine.

A GP with special skills may also be willing to undertake simple treatments, in particular aiding ovulation where appropriate, with the drug clomiphene. However, in most cases, further tests and treatment will need a referral to an infertility specialist.

Further tests that can help to pin-point exactly where the problem lies include:

➤ a post-coital test, to see how well sperm penetrate through the cervical mucus. This involves taking a small sample of mucus, around the time of ovulation, and within twelve hours of intercourse

➤ a series of ultrasound scans can see if any follicles (small lumps containing eggs) develop in the ovaries during the course of a month, and whether ovulation takes place

➤ a hysterosalpingogram (HSG) is a special X-ray of the womb and Fallopian tubes. X-ray visible dye is injected through the cervix and passes up through the womb and into the Fallopian tubes. Any blockage or abnormality prevents passage of the dye. This procedure is usually done without an anaesthetic, and though it's not painful, it can be slightly uncomfortable

➤ a laparoscopy (see page 118) can be done to inspect all the pelvic organs, and it's common for a dye test to be done at the same time (this is when a special blue dye, inserted through the cervix, can be seen to fill, then spill, from open Fallopian tubes).

Treatments

Treatment should always be geared to the underlying problem.

Hostile cervical mucus, which is too thick to allow sperm to penetrate, can be by-passed by injecting a sample of semen directly into the womb. Known as AIH (Artificial Insemination with Husband's semen), it can be a relatively easy and successful route to a pregnancy. A similar procedure, AID (Artificial Insemination by Donor), which uses donor semen, can be used as a way for a women to have a child when her regular partner has a poor sperm count.

There are several different types of drugs available that can help ovulation problems.

Clomiphene boosts the levels of the hormone FSH, which in turn stimulates the ovaries. Though it can sometimes cause two eggs to be released, and therefore increase the risk of twins, over-stimulation and the release of several eggs is relatively rare. It's usually given as just five tablets to be taken at the beginning of each period. There is a slight increased risk of ovarian cancer with this drug.

Human Menopausal gonadotrophin, or HMG, contains a concentrated mixture of FSH and LH. It's a powerful drug, given by injection, which stimulates the ovaries directly. It can result in the development of several eggs at once. Anyone given HMG should be very carefully monitored by regular ultrasound scans. It can easily over-stimulate the ovaries, and carries at least a 30 percent risk of a multiple pregnancy. It can also have serious side-effects, including the development of large ovarian cysts. As soon as over-stimulation of the ovaries is suspected, treatment should be stopped immediately.

LHRH is a hormone that stimulates the pituitary gland to release the hormones FSH and LH, which in turn stimulate the ovaries (see page 119). LHRH is normally produced in short pulses by the brain, and this can be mimicked by injecting the drug at regular intervals via a special syringe driver. This type of treatment (which is only available in very specialized centres) can be helpful for women with very low natural hormone levels, and for women with polycystic ovaries.

In the past, tubal surgery was used to try and correct blocked Fallopian tubes. Overall, however, results from tubal surgery are very disappointing, and even if the tubes are cleared, they remain scarred. Pregnancy rates after tubal surgery are generally very low, and there's also an increased risk of an ectopic pregnancy occurring. Nowadays, most specialists only operate on very slightly damaged tubes. For the others, IVF usually offers a far greater chance of a successful pregnancy.

IN-VITRO FERTILISATION (IVF)

This is the 'test-tube baby' method. It's increasingly used for women with blocked tubes, and for couples who have 'unexplained' infertility. A special variation of the technique, ICSI, can be used to treat male infertility.

Despite it's increasing popularity, IVF success rates are still disappointingly low. Even in the best clinics and in young women in their mid-twenties, the chances of success are only about 30 percent. For women in their thirties, this figure is sadly much lower.

It involves stimulating the development of as many as twelve eggs at once inside the ovaries, using a combination of different hormones usually given by nasal spray and injections. The drugs given can slightly increase the risk of developing ovarian cancer. Once the eggs are 'ripe' they have to be collected, either through a laparoscope, or through the top of the vagina, under ultrasound guidance.

The eggs are then mixed in the laboratory, with a specially prepared sample of fresh sperm. Up to three fertilized eggs, or embryos, are then carefully replaced back in the womb, usually two to three days later. Any remaining embryos may be frozen, and kept at the hospital for later use.

The method can fail at any stage. In some women, the drugs fail to stimulate the growth of any egg-containing follicles inside the ovaries. Sometimes, none of the eggs are fertilized by the sperm, or the eggs that do fertilize form very poor quality embryos, which don't survive. More common than either of these is a failure of the embryos to implant in the womb. And even if IVF does appear to be initially successful, the miscarriage rate is higher than in normal pregnancies. Even in the safest hands, and with close monitoring, the drugs used in IVF can overstimulate the ovaries and lead to the development of large ovarian cysts, and severe abdominal pain.

IVF involves a huge time and emotional commitment. It also tends to involve a large financial commitment as well. In some areas of the country it's possible to have one attempt funded by the NHS, but most couples will have to fund IVF themselves. Even if you are self-funding, it may be possible to obtain the drugs needed on an NHS prescription from your GP – which can mean a saving of £500 or more. IVF costs vary enormously. Treatment centres attached to NHS hospitals often offer cheaper rates than completely private clinics. Results vary enormously too. If you are considering IVF it's vital to 'shop around'. All good units should be happy to give you a list of their results for the different age groups of women treated. Look at these carefully, and if necessary, ask your GP to help with their interpretation. The statistic that's all important is not the pregnancy rate, but the 'take-home baby rate'. This is exactly what it says – the percentage of women undergoing IVF who eventually have a live baby to take home.

GIFT is a variation of IVF. However, instead of mixing the eggs and sperm in a test tube, they are placed together directly into the Fallopian tube. Overall success rates are not any better than normal IVF, and some centres are phasing it out as a method of treatment.

In women who have had a premature menopause or who do not produce any healthy eggs of their own, IVF can be performed using eggs donated by another woman. Once the eggs are fertilized, they can be placed in the womb of the infertile woman (which has been prepared first by hormonal treatment). This allows infertile women to have the pleasure and responsibility of their own pregnancy and birth.

Sadly, there is a desperate shortage of donor eggs in this country. Unlike donating sperm, donating eggs requires a time commitment, and can carry risks. Donors have to be prepared to have the usual fertility drugs to stimulate their ovaries into producing several eggs at once, and then undergo an egg retrieval procedure.

TREATMENTS FOR MALE INFERTILITY
In the past, treating male infertility has been a rather neglected area. However, progress is now being made and new treatments are becoming available that can offer real hope to men with abnormal sperm counts.
➤ If low hormone levels are to blame, regular injections with either the hormone HCG or HMG may help. In some men, pump treatment with LHRH (like that used in women) can improve sperm production.
➤ Treating infections with appropriate antibiotics can help to clear debris from semen, thus improving sperm mobility.
➤ Some men are infertile because they develop antibodies against their own sperm. This can sometimes be successfully treated using high-dose steroids, but IVF, using specially 'washed' sperm, often gives better results.
➤ Structural defects affecting sperm production, such as dilated veins around the testis (a varicocele), or water around the testis (a hydrocele) can be treated surgically.
With all theses treatments, the improvement in the sperm count is not immediate – it's usually only apparant three to six months later.

INTRA-CYTOPLASMIC SPERM INJECTION (ICSI)
This is a specialised form of IVF that can be used as a treatment for male infertility. Instead of mixing the eggs with the sperm in a test tube, a single active, healthy-looking sperm is isolated, and injected directly into the egg. Though it's technically difficult, it's proving increasingly successful as a treatment for men with either a very low sperm count, or those with a proportion of abnormal sperm. For ICSI, a single sperm IS enough! It may also soon be possible to use sperm taken directly, through a needle, from the tubes surrounding the testis, rather than from an ejaculated sample. This will overcome problems caused by an anatomical blockage in any part of the male genital tract.

Facing up to infertility
Having a child is, for many women, one of the most important aims in life, and the thought that this might not happen can be absolutely devastating.

Although going to an infertility clinic can be viewed as a positive step towards solving an infertility problem, it can also be very frightening. Even minor tests can become hugely important, and it's all too easy to let infertility take over your life.

Infertility can be like a treadmill – once you start investigations and treatment it can be difficult to know when to stop. One test soon leads to another, then another, and before you realize it all your activities revolve around hospital appointments, and trying to get pregnant. Many previously secure relationships crumble under the strain. At each stage, it's important to take stock with your partner, and think just how much of your time and your emotions you are prepared to commit to your pursuit of trying to have a baby. If it's all getting too much, then say so. Don't be too scared to tell your doctors you need a break from it all. Don't worry about their reactions – they will almost certainly respect your honesty, and be prepared to see you again when you feel ready.

IVF can cause an almost intolerable emotional strain. It can be difficult to carry on with normal day-to-day life when a daily injection, combined with frequent hospital visits, are constant reminders of what you are trying to achieve. Many couples find the two week wait after embryo transfer almost unbearable, and feel near to absolute despair if a period then begins.

There is no easy way to cope with infertility, but it is important to try and avoid letting it rule your life. Don't sit at home and brood. Many relationships fall apart because the partner with the problem feels guilty and inadequate. Talk things through, and if necesary, go and see a counsellor. Most infertility units can now arrange this for you.

Preventing infertility
Infertility is often unavoidable, and no one should blame themselves, or others, for a fertility problem. However, there are steps you can take that can help reduce the risks of some causes of infertility:
➤ don't delay any longer than you really need to before trying for a baby. A woman's fertility falls dramatically in her mid-thirties, and waiting till your career is well established may be a little too late for your biological clock
➤ don't be promiscuous. The greater the number of sexual partners you have, the greater your chance of acquiring a sexually transmitted infection, that could damage your fallopian tubes
➤ use barrier contraceptives, especially for the first few months of any new relationship, to avoid acquiring a sexually transmitted disease which could damage your Fallopian tubes

➤ seek prompt medical help for a vaginal discharge that might be sexually transmitted, or for other symptoms that might indicate an infection, such as pelvic pain, or pain during intercourse

➤ avoid using an IUCD for contraception, preferably until you are settled in a relationship and have had at least one child.

IRRITABLE BOWEL SYNDROME

Up to one in five people suffer from Irritable Bowel Syndrome (IBS). It's twice as common in women than men. Symptoms include:

➤ intermittent cramp-like abdominal pain. This is often felt on the left hand side, but can occur anywhere

➤ erratic bowel motions, with typically bouts of diarrhoea, interspersed with hard motions or constipation

➤ a bloated feeling, belching, and the passing of large amounts of wind (which may smell awful)

➤ passing mucus with motions (but not blood)

➤ a feeling that you need to empty your bowels just after you've been to the toilet.

Many people who suffer from IBS also admit to frequent bouts of nausea, tiredness and headaches. Symptoms vary from person to person, and may last anything from a few days to a few weeks.

It's thought to be caused by abnormal contractions of the muscles that move food waste along inside the large intestine. The reason this occurs is often a mystery, but stress and anxiety are common triggers. Certain foods which may irritate the bowel lining in sensitive people, may also be to blame.

Self-help

In many cases, self-help measures really can help to either prevent, or ease, IBS.

➤ Try to reduce the stress in your life. Make sure you have some relaxation time each day, and that you get enough sleep. Being overtired always makes IBS worse.

➤ Aromatherapy, massage and yoga can help to relieve stress and tension. Some patients have also found hypnosis useful.

➤ Take regular exercise – a little every day is better than a vigorous burst once a week (though this is better than none at all).

➤ Keep a food diary to see if you can identify any food triggers. Common culprits are large amounts of diary produce, spicy foods and large quantities of pulses.

➤ Avoid eating too much fibre. A reasonable amount is necessary to prevent constipation, but excessive amounts often lead to bloating and wind.

➤ Avoid huge meals. Eating little and often is best, with a diet that includes five small helpings of fresh fruit and vegetables each day, and one that's low in fats and sugar.

➤ Drink plenty of good-quality water and avoid carbonated drinks, tea and coffee which can all irritate the bowel lining.

Help from your doctor

If symptoms persist despite these measures, then it's important to see your doctor. It's important to be sure that you do have IBS and not a more serious bowel condition. Further investigations, such as a barium X-ray of your bowel, may be necessary.

Prescription drugs available for IBS include peppermint oil capsules, which can relieve pain and bloating and muscle relaxants, such as dicyclomine. These are useful for relieving pain and diarrhoea. If constipation is a problem, bulking agents such as Fybogel may help, and capsules such as loperamide can help to stop very loose stools.

For best effect a combination of drugs may be required. They don't necessarily need to be taken all the time, but can be taken on an 'as necessary ' basis, according to symptoms.

L

LABIA

This is the proper name for the folds of skin surrounding the entrance to the vagina and the opening of the urethra (which leads up to the bladder). There are two pairs of labia on each side of the vagina. The outer pair, the labia majora, are thick and fleshy, and contain sweat glands. The inner pair, the labia minora, are narrow and wrinkled and are of variable depth. In some women they are so long that they can interfere with lovemaking, in which case, the size can be reduced by a simple operation. The labia can become inflamed from infections such as thrush and herpes, and from skin conditions, such as eczema.

LAPAROSCOPY

This is a method of examining and operating on internal organs, using a special telescope, or laparoscope, while the patient is under a general anaesthetic. Gynaecologists have been using laparoscopes for many years to look at the pelvic organs; to diagnose conditions such as endometriosis and pelvic inflammatory disease (PID); and to perform sterilization procedures. In the last few years, laparoscopes have been used for far more complex operations, such as hysterectomies, removing the gall bladder or appendix, and hernia repairs. Compared to conventional surgery, laparoscopic or keyhole surgery, usually means a much smaller scar; less pain; a shorter stay in hospital; a reduced risk of infection; and a much quicker return to normal activity. However, laparoscopic surgery can be technically much more difficult than a conventional operation, and mistakes do occur. Any patient offered, or considering laparoscopic surgery, should make sure that their surgeon has undergone special keyhole surgery training and is experienced in this type of work (see Useful Addresses).

What's involved?

To begin with, about three litres of carbon dioxide gas is pumped into the abdominal cavity to inflate the stomach and to separate the internal organs. Though much of this gas is removed at the end of the operation, it can cause a bloated feeling afterwards and an ache around the chest and shoulders.

Next the laparoscope is inserted through a small hole, about an inch long, which is made just below the tummy button. Additional small instruments, such as probes (which look like long skewers), may be inserted through additional tiny cuts elsewhere on the tummy wall. Several of these cuts may be needed for complex operations, such as gall bladder removal. A simple gynaecological laparoscopy usually only takes about fifteen minutes, and it's normal to go home the same day. Patients having more major surgery usually need to stay in hospital for a further two or three days. It's normal to feel tired and uncomfortable for a few days afterwards, and it's advisable to have help around the house, and to stay off work, for at least a week.

LH–RH

This is the abbreviation for Luteinizing Hormone Releasing Hormone. It's produced by a part of the brain called the hypothalamus, and it stimulates the pituitary gland to secrete the hormones FSH and LH. Synthetic LHRH is now used increasingly for treating infertility and other gynaecological disorders. Injections at carefully timed ninety minute intervals (via a battery-driven portable pump) can stimulate ovulation. Giving larger doses at less frequent intervals has the opposite effect, switching off ovulation and the menstrual cycle. It's an effective treatment for endometriosis, and can also be used to shrink fibroids prior to surgery. It's also used to 'turn off' the natural ovarian cycle as part of the complicated drug regime used in IVF.

LIBIDO

(see Sexual Problems page 153).

LUPUS

Otherwise known as systemic lupus erythematosis, or SLE, this is an auto-immune disorder whereby the body's own immune system attacks numerous body tissues, including the joints, the kidneys, heart, lungs and skin. It's nine times more common in women than men, and can cause recurrent miscarriages.

Treatment is with powerful anti-inflammatory drugs. The severity of the illness can vary enormously, and although it can be fatal, many women live for years with only moderate symptoms. A milder form of the illness, discoid lupus, affects exposed areas of skin only.

M

THE MENOPAUSE

This is the time in a woman's life when her ovaries cease to function. In effect, this means that ovulation no longer occurs, and the ovaries are no longer able to produce the hormone oestrogen. This normally occurs between the ages of forty-nine and fifty-one, but it can be much earlier or later than this.

An early menopause can occur spontaneously, or it can be induced by either surgically removing the ovaries; by radiotherapy to the pelvis; or by some forms of chemotherapy.

The most obvious, and for many women the only, sign of the menopause is that monthly periods stop completely. This may occur abruptly, or they may be erratic for several months beforehand.

A lot of women sail through the menopause with no problems at all, and seem to be completely unaffected by it. For others, it's a time of great physical and emotional disturbance. Erratic periods in women in their forties aren't always due to the menopause – sometimes gaps occur and then regular periods start up again. A simple blood test, which your GP can arrange, can give an accurate diagnosis, and show whether you are menopausal or not. It can also indicate if you are likely to become menopausal in the near future.

MENOPAUSAL 'MYTHS'

➤ 'Everyone suffers.' No they don't. At least 50 percent of women don't have hot flushes or sweats.

➤ 'It's the start of old age.' No it's not. Ageing is a gradual process. In fact, some women get a new lease of life when they no longer have to worry about monthly periods or accidental pregnancy.

➤ 'It means putting on weight.' Your metabolic rate does fall gradually with increasing age – and in practice that means that if you eat the same in your fifties as you did in your twenties you will put on weight. But there's no sudden change at the menopause. If you're careful with your diet, and take plenty of exercise, your weight should stay the same.

➤ 'It goes on for years.' No, it doesn't. The menopause itself only last a few months at the most – but the effects of lack of oestrogen may be felt for years.

SYMPTOMS
It's the plummeting oestrogen levels that are responsible for the symptoms many women suffer from during this time. The first of these may start before periods actually stop. These include:
➤ hot flushes and sweats, which can occur at any time but are often worse at night. These can continue anything from a few weeks to a couple of years
➤ headaches, mood swings, irritability, difficulty sleeping and depression.
After a few months, other symptoms can appear. These include:
➤ a dry vagina, which is occasionally sore and itchy, making sex uncomfortable
➤ frequent bouts of cystitis
➤ loss of libido
➤ thinning skin
➤ joint aches and pains.
Later on, after several years, low oestrogen levels have two other very important health effects. These are
➤ thin bones, or osteoporosis. (see page 128)
➤ an increased risk of heart disease due to thickening and hardening of the lining of the coronary arteries.
Sadly, neither of these tends to cause any symptoms until they are well advanced, and difficult to treat. That's why prevention is so important.

M

Self-help
You can reduce the effects of hot flushes and sweats by:
➤ wearing several layers of light clothing, rather than one thick layer. That way, you can shed a layer when you need to
➤ cut down on caffeine, alcohol and cigarettes, which can widen blood vessels and make flushes worse
➤ avoid steaming hot baths. Have a warm shower instead
➤ use a lubricating jelly, such as K-Y, to make sex more comfortable
➤ eat a low-fat healthy diet with plenty of fresh fruit and vegetables, to help keep your heart healthy (see page 180)
➤ regular weight-bearing exercise and at least 1,000mg of calcium a day can help to keep bones strong
➤ make sure your supplement includes magnesium, which helps to direct calcium to the bones rather than the soft tissues of the body.

➤ wearing clothes made of cotton and other natural fabrics, which allow your skin to breathe. Avoid synthetics, such as nylon and polyester, as much as possible

Help from your doctor
Hormone Replacement Therapy (HRT) can ease both the unpleasant symptoms of the menopause, such as flushes and sweats, and help to prevent the long-term effects of a low oestrogen level, particularly osteoporosis and heart disease. See page 96 for more details.

Drugs that don't contain hormones, such as clonidine, can help to ease flushes and sweats. Oestrogen creams and pessaries can be used inside the vagina to ease any dryness and itching.

If you find it difficult to adjust to the menopause, counselling may be of help.

METABOLISM
This is the rate at which the body burns up calories to provide energy for normal body functions. It's controlled by various hormones, including the thyroid hormone, insulin, and adrenaline. Metabolism can vary between people. Those with a high metabolic rate can eat a lot of calorie-laden food without gaining weight, while others with a naturally lower metabolism put on weight very easily.

Your basic metabolic rate falls with increasing age. On average a young women of twenty requires 2,200 calories each day for normal activities, but a woman of fifty requires only 1,500 – that's a third less. Eating the same throughout life, with no adjustments, is the main reason for the appearance of middle age spread! Larger women have slightly higher calorie requirements than smaller women – one reason why continued weight loss can be difficult if you're on a successful diet, as the metabolic rate falls slightly as you get slimmer.

The best way to boost your metabolic rate is by exercise. Women who exercise not only burn calories during the activity, but their metabolic rate stays raised for some time afterwards. The more often and vigorously you exercise, the greater the effect.

MISCARRIAGE
It's thought that as many as one in four pregnancies end in a miscarriage. This figure isn't clear cut because until recently many women who had miscarriages weren't sure that they were pregnant, and assumed that they were having a late, heavy period. However,

modern pregnancy tests, easily available from chemists, mean that it's possible to diagnose a pregnancy from the first day of a missed period, and it's becoming clear that many babies are lost in the first few weeks following fertilization.

The majority of miscarriages occur in the first twelve weeks of pregnancy. In many cases it's because the baby just isn't developing normally – either the sperm or the egg were defective to begin with, or they didn't fuse properly. A miscarriage can be regarded as nature's way of dealing with its mistakes – and preventing a very handicapped baby. In many of these cases the baby stops growing and dies, approximately six weeks after fertilization, but the tell-tale bleeding may not occur until two or three weeks later. Sometimes the baby never forms at all.

Other causes of miscarriage include any severe illness, particularly one that causes a high fever. Some viral illnesses, such as rubella and Cyto-Megalo virus (CMV), which can cause foetal abnormalities, can also cause miscarriage. Less commonly, miscarriage can be due to hormonal problems, such as a deficiency in progesterone secretion, or chronic illness, such as SLE (see Lupus, page 119).

Slightly later on in pregnancy, a miscarriage can be caused by an abnormality in the womb, such as fibroids, which interfere with the growth of the baby. A weak cervix, which may have been caused by damage to the muscle fibres during a previous termination, may also be to blame.

The first sign of a miscarriage is usually vaginal bleeding, which can be very heavy, with the passage of large clots. In addition there is usually severe, cramp-like lower abdominal pain. In many cases, the diagnosis is clear, but if there is any doubt as to whether the baby is still alive, an ultrasound scan should be performed.

It's important that the womb is completely emptied after a miscarriage. Any remaining fragments of tissue can easily become infected, causing heavy bleeding, pain and possible pelvic scarring. In very early miscarriages, complete emptying may occur spontaneously, but later on an ERPC operation (evacuation of the retained products of conception) is usually required. This is similar to a D and C (see page 51).

Miscarriage is a very common event, and most women who have suffered one go on to have a normal pregnancy without any difficulties. Even for women who've had two miscarriages, there's a 70 percent chance of success the next time they try. But women who have had three or more miscarriages in a row should consider having investigations to see if there's a treatable cause.

A miscarriage is always a very upsetting physical and emotional experience. Afterwards, it's important to give yourself time to recover. It's normal to feel tired and drained, and the sudden drop in hormones can add to the inevitable depression that follows the loss of a baby. Though you may want to try and get pregnant again as soon as possible, it's best to wait until at you've had at least one period, which normally occurs four to six weeks after the miscarriage.

Self-help
In the majority of cases a miscarriage is just a very sad quirk of nature. It's no-one's fault and nothing could have prevented it. But you can take some positive steps to try and improve your chances of a successful pregnancy next time.
➤ Concentrate on a really healthy lifestyle. Stop smoking (which can increase the risk of a miscarriage occurring), reduce your alcohol intake, and aim for a balanced diet with plenty of fresh fruit and vegetables.
➤ Take a folic acid supplement of 0.4mg each day to help prevent spina bifida and other brain and spinal cord defects.
➤ Avoid taking any other unnecessary supplements or medications. This includes herbal preparations, especially penny royal, tansy, mugwort and slippery elm, which may increase the risk of miscarriage.
Remember that it takes two to make a healthy baby, so tackle your partners lifestyle in the same way. Stopping smoking and cutting down on alcohol are particularly important in men.

See Useful Addresses (page 189) for a list of useful organisations.

MYALGIC ENCEPHALITIS (M.E.)

Also known as Chronic Fatigue Syndrome, M.E. can cause a variety of symptoms, but the most prominent is always severe muscle fatigue and exhaustion. Any mental or physical effort, particularly physical exercise, tends to make this worse, and the tiredness is not usually relieved by sleep. Other symptoms can include generalized muscle and joint pains, memory lapses, a loss of concentration, and digestive problems. Many sufferers are also very depressed.

In some cases the illness follows on from a viral infection, but in many cases there is no obvious cause. Some doctors consider that it is an unusual and severe form of depression.There is no specific treatment available, although many sufferers are helped by anti-depressant tablets. Others find stress management, graded exercise, special diets with vitamin and mineral supplements helpful. Although a few people continue to suffer for many years, most people with ME do eventually make a full recovery.

MULTIPLE SCLEROSIS

This is a disease of the central nervous system. The sheaths of myelin, which protect and surround the nerves of the brain and spinal cord, are destroyed in a random and patchy way, preventing the passage of nerve impulses. The reason this occurs is not known – it is thought to be partly due to an abnormal reaction to the body's own immune system, possibly as a result of a viral infection earlier in life.

The first symptoms of MS usually appear between the ages of twenty and forty. It is slightly more common in women than men and in the UK approximately 2,400 new cases occur each year.

Symptoms

In most patients, the onset of the disease is signalled by one main symptom. This can be:
➤ leg weakness
➤ a painful eye and blurred vision
➤ a tingling sensation in either an arm or a leg.
Other symptoms can include:
➤ unsteady walking
➤ facial pain
➤ bladder problems.
MS is a very unpredictable illness. Some patients only have occasional attacks of symptoms from which they make a nearly full recovery. Others have frequent attacks, which gradually cause severe disability over a period of months or years. There is no single test that can confirm MS – the diagnosis is made by excluding other conditions using specialized nerve and brain tests.

As yet, there is no curative treatment. Some patients have felt that they have benefitted from special diets, or from taking evening primrose oil supplements, but in many others there is no difference at all. Steroids are often used during acute relapses to try and prevent serious damage to the nerves by inflammation. Recently, the drug interferon beta-1b has been shown to reduce the number of acute relapses in some patients and may help to prevent the disease progressing, but unfortunately it is very expensive, and again, in some patients, it is no benefit at all.

N

NAILS

Healthy nails are slightly rounded, pale pink, shiny and smooth. They are made up of dead skin cells that harden to form a tough protein called keratin. Finger nails grow at the rate of an eighth of inch a month, although this does speed up slightly in hot weather (and slows down in the winter). Nail growth also speeds up during pregnancy, and just before a period! This means that it takes about six months for finger nails to grow from base to tip. Toe nails grow a quarter of an inch every four months. This means that any injury to a toe nail can take a year to grow out!

Like all parts of the body, a healthy diet is essential for strong healthy nails. Going on a crash diet will slow down nail growth, and serious illness can have a similar effect. Eating extra calcium or gelatin won't help to strengthen your nails.

Split, weak nails are often simply caused by housework. Constantly immersing them in water weakens the keratin, and exposure to household detergents makes the problem worse. Weak nails can also be due to overuse of nail-hardening products and nail varnish removers, which can strip nails of their natural moisture. Occasionally, split nails can be a sign of an underactive thyroid gland (see page 166).

Horizontal ridges across nails are often a sign of trauma, especially over-enthusiastic manicuring of the cuticles. It can also be a sign of slower nail growth due to dieting or illness. White flecks are also a sign of trauma, and are often seen in people who chew their nails.

Weak nails that separate easily from the nail bed can be caused by repeatedly immersing them in water, but it can also be a sign of a fungal infection. Fungal infections can also cause thickened, flaky nails that have a yellow discolouration – this is a particularly common problem affecting toe nails. Small pits in the nails are often linked with the skin condition psoriasis.

Ingrowing toe nails are caused by incorrect cutting (curving the scissors round the sides) together with wearing tight pointed shoes. The area around the side of the nail often becomes infected, forming a blister of pus (a whitlow). Although antibiotics may help to cure this in the early stages, often the only way to clear the infection is to surgically remove the ingrowing piece of nail.

Self-help for strong nails
➤ Keep them out of water as much as possible. Wear cotton-lined rubber gloves for all types of housework and cleaning, even if you're only washing up a couple of coffee cups!
➤ Keep your nails relatively short. Long nails are more prone to splits and breaks. File them after a bath or a shower, when they're slightly softer, and less likely to split.
➤ Apply a moisturizing cream at least twice a day, rubbing it in well around the nail bed. Do this all the year round to your toes as well as your hands. For presentable toes in the summer, you need to take action in the middle of winter!
➤ Be gentle on your nails, especially the cuticles. Avoid using metal manicure instruments – use a rubber-ended hoof stick instead.
➤ Only wear nail varnish occasionally. Although varnishes containing nylon fibres may help to protect fragile nails, varnish removers can be very drying, and should be used no more than once a week. It's better to touch-up chipped varnish than to strip it off the whole nail and start again.
➤ Cut toe nails straight across, with only a very slight curve at the corners. Never dig the scissors down the sides!

Help from your doctor
➤ Fungal infections can be diagnosed by an analysis of nail clippings. These infections used to be very difficult to treat but new paints, such as Tioconazole and Terbinafine tablets, are proving very successful (although six months' treatment may be required for a cure). They are only available on prescription.
➤ See your doctor as soon as possible if you develop redness and soreness around the side of a toe nail. Early treatment with antibiotics may save you painful surgical treatment!

NIPPLES
(see under Breasts page 26).

O

ORGASM

This is the name for a sexual climax. In women it causes rhythmic contractions of the pelvic floor muscles, the vagina and the clitoris, usually accompanied by an intense feeling of pleasure and a release of tension. The intensity of orgasms can vary enormously. Unlike men, many women are able to have multiple orgasms, one after another.

Most women need some sort of direct stimulation of the clitoris to reach an orgasm. Though there is a very sensitive area on the front wall of the vagina (the G spot), stimulation of this alone is rarely sufficient for an orgasm to occur. This means that in practice it's often difficult for a woman to have a simultaneous orgasm with her partner during ordinary intercourse. Manually stimulating the clitoris at the same time can often make simultaneous orgasms a bit easier. Women usually need a great deal more stimulation to reach an orgasm than men. It's a sign of a good relationship if you are able to teach your partner the best way to stimulate, and satisfy, your sexual needs.

It also takes time for you to learn what type of stimulation you enjoy, and then to teach your partner how to please you. However, there's far more to enjoyable sex than orgasms, and no women should feel pressurized into feeling she has 'to come' (and then end up faking it!). Many women find the sexual experience of physical closeness, hugging, kissing and satisfying their partner every bit as pleasurable as an orgasm.

OSTEOPOROSIS

Osteoporosis is a condition whereby bones become thin and fragile. Unfortunately, some degree of osteoporosis is a natural part of ageing. A woman's bones reach their maximum density in her mid-thirties, and then gradually become thinner. The hormone oestrogen helps to keep bones strong, and at the menopause, when hormone levels fall dramatically, bone loss increases. It's a silent process, and in the early stages osteoporosis causes no symptoms. Many women discover they have osteoporosis by chance when they break a bone, typically a wrist or the top of the leg, near the hip, after a trivial fall.

In the more advanced stages, osteoporosis causes loss of height and a curved spine (the classic 'dowager's hump'), due to thinner bones in the back, which gradually become crushed and wedge shaped.

Unfortunately, osteoporosis is nearly always a permanent condition – once bones become thin there's little that can be done to make them strong again. Although men do suffer from osteoporosis, the condition is far more common in women, who have naturally thinner bones.

Some women are at particular risk of developing osteoporosis. These include:

➤ thin women, especially those with a small frame
➤ women who have poor nutrition, or who have suffered from anorexia (especially if periods stopped because of low body weight)
➤ smokers
➤ those treated with steroid tablets
➤ alcohol abusers
➤ women who have prolonged inactivity
➤ women who have had an early menopause or their ovaries removed before the age of forty-five.

Significant osteoporosis is more common in women over sixty, and a quarter of women above this age suffer a fracture of the wrist or hip as a result. But this can occur at a much younger age, and some women in their mid-twenties are affected. Although bones can appear thin on an ordinary X-ray, osteoporosis is best diagnosed by a bone density scan. This can either be arranged directly through your GP, or via a specialist hospital clinic.

Because osteoporosis is so difficult to treat, prevention is vitally important for all women, and surprisingly easy!

Self-help to prevent osteoporosis
The best way to prevent osteoporosis is to build strong bones during childhood and adolescence. But it's never too late to start.

➤ Eat plenty of calcium, preferably at least 1000mg a day. Good sources are dairy produce, oily fish, and green leafy vegetables.
➤ Boost your intake if necessary with a daily tablet supplement, but make sure that it includes magnesium for good calcium absorption into the bones.
➤ Take regular exercise. Weight-bearing exercise is best, such as walking, running, tennis or badminton, but any exercise is better than none at all! Aim to do at least half an hour, three times a week. But beware of overdoing it – athletes who train so much that their periods stop are at increased risk of osteoporosis.

➤ Drink no more than fourteen units of alcohol weekly.
➤ Don't smoke.
➤ Consider taking hormone-replacement therapy (HRT) as soon as your periods stop (or immediately after an operation to remove the ovaries).

Treatment
Once the bones are thin, the main aim of treatment is preventing further bone loss.
This can be achieved by:
➤ HRT in post-menopausal women. The dose is important – some low-dose formulations may not give maximum bone protection. The best way to check the dose you are receiving is by an oestradiol blood test. There is some evidence that higher doses of HRT may help to build new bone
➤ eating plenty of calcium – preferably 1000mg daily together with magnesium
➤ taking plenty of weight-bearing exercise
➤ Etidronate and alendronate are relatively new drugs that prevent further bone loss, and like HRT may help to build new bone. They are available on prescription only.

OVARIES
Each women normally has a pair of ovaries situated just below the open end of the Fallopian tube, on each side of the pelvis. Each ovary is almond shaped, approximately 3cm long and 2cm wide. In adult women the ovaries secrete the hormones oestrogen and progesterone, together with a small amount of the male hormone testosterone. Inside each ovary are numerous tiny follicles, each of which contains an immature egg. A woman is born with her full quota of eggs, usually around a million immature eggs. Only approximately 400 of these eggs mature and are released. The rest slowly shrivel away, and by the time of the menopause there are none left. The eggs are more prone to defects with increasing age – which is why older mums are more at risk of having a baby with Down's syndrome, or other congenital abnormalities.

Approximately once a month a follicle in one of the ovaries swells, and releases the egg, or ovum. Each egg is approximately 0.1mm in diameter, much larger than a sperm. Occasionally more than one egg is released, and if they are both fertilized, this can result in non-identical twins (or triplets if three eggs are released).

Occasionally ovaries become inflamed from pelvic inflammatory disease (PID), or affected by endometriosis, and have to be removed. Most women can function normally with only one ovary, which produces an egg each month and enough hormones to compensate for the loss of the other one. It's also possible to get pregnant without difficulty with only one ovary. However, removal of both ovaries – a bilateral oophorectomy – does automatically mean an instant loss of fertility, and in younger women who are ovulating, an instant menopause. All women under forty-five who have both ovaries removed should consider taking hormone-replacement therapy (HRT) to prevent osteoporosis and heart disease (see page 96).

OVARIAN CYSTS

Fluid-filled sacs can develop in the ovaries at any age. In the vast majority of cases they are benign – that is, non cancerous. Taking the combined contraceptive pill helps to prevent ovarian cysts. Small cysts often form from developing egg follicles, and many of these disappear of their own accord. However, some ovarian cysts can grow to a vast size. Many cysts contain just fluid, but others may contain structures such as hair, bone and even teeth – these are called dermoid cysts.

Many ovarian cysts produce no symptoms and are only discovered at a routine pelvic examination. However, they can twist or rupture, causing acute, severe abdominal pain. Some can cause vague lower abdominal discomfort, which is worse during sex. Some cysts produce hormones and cause irregular periods. Larger cysts can cause a noticeable bulge in the lower tummy wall.

Although cysts can often be suspected during a pelvic examination by an experienced doctor, an ultrasound scan is necessary for a definite diagnosis. Immediate treatment isn't always necessary, as many very small cysts will go away of their own accord, but larger cysts should always be removed, especially if there is a suspicion (from the ultrasound scan) that a cyst may be cancerous. Surgically it's often possible to remove just the cyst and the ovarian tissue that's left behind usually continues to function normally. Removing larger cysts, however, often involves removing the whole ovary.

Polycystic ovarian syndrome is a relatively common condition where multiple small cysts develop in the ovaries, and are linked with a hormone imbalance. See page 144.

OVARIAN CANCER

Ovarian cancer can occur at any age, but is more common in older women aged fifty to sixty. It is more common in women who have never had children, and in those who have had drug treatment to induce ovulation as an infertility treatment. This includes women who have taken clomiphene as well as those who have had IVF. It can also run in families, and if your mother or sister had ovarian cancer then you are at slightly increased risk. The risk is greatly increased if several close family members have been affected, or have had breast, womb or colon cancer. The combined contraceptive pill, however, can help to reduce the risk of developing ovarian cancer by as much as 50 percent (see page 69).

Though ovarian cancer may cause vague pelvic discomfort, sadly it often produces no symptoms at all until it has reached quite an advanced stage, and spread from the affected ovary. Even then the only symptom may be a vague feeling of fullness or bloating. Later on it can cause loss of appetite, more noticeable pelvic discomfort, nausea and vomiting.

Once the diagnosis is suspected, an ultrasound scan can confirm an ovarian cyst or mass, and can often indicate whether it is likely to be cancerous. However, the diagnosis can only be confirmed by directly examining the ovary and removing the cyst. If cancer is confirmed, both ovaries, and the womb, should be removed. Depending on the extent of the tumour, chemotherapy, and occasionally radiotherapy, is given afterwards.

If the cancer is confined to the ovaries, the chance of surviving more than five years is over 90 percent. However, this falls to 50 percent if the cancer has spread to the other pelvic organs.

Self-help

As with all cancers, the earlier ovarian cancer is detected the greater the chance of an effective cure.

All women should have a pelvic examination at least once every three years – usually at the same time as a cervical smear. This is particularly important for women who have had infertility treatment and are at slightly higher risk.

Women with a family history of ovarian cancer should have more intensive screening, preferably in the form of an ultrasound scan, at least once every three years. A measurement of the blood level of the chemical CA125, which rises in ovarian cancer, may also be helpful for these women.

PANIC ATTACKS

Everyone has felt fear at some time in their life, but it normally occurs as part of a normal reaction to a nasty event. A panic attack is a sudden, intense feeling of fear, which usually occurs out of the blue, for no apparent reason. Panic attacks cause physical symptoms, which can include:

➤ breathing problems, varying from breathing very fast, to a feeling of intense tightness in the chest
➤ dizziness
➤ palpitations and sweating
➤ tingling in the fingers and toes
➤ shaking and trembling.

Panic attacks are often brought on by stress. This can either be due to a sudden event, such as a bereavement, or redundancy, or more long-term stress, such as ongoing marital or money worries. They are twice as common in women than men.

Self-help

Many of the nasty physical effects of a panic attack, such as tingling and dizziness, are caused by breathing too fast, and taking breaths that are too shallow (hyperventilating), which can reduce the carbon dioxide level in the blood stream to an abnormally low level.

As soon as you feel a panic attack starting, take action.

➤ Concentrate really hard on taking long, slow, deep breaths.
➤ Covering your nose and mouth with a paper bag will help even more, as this quickly raise the carbon dioxide level in the blood back to normal. (It must be a PAPER bag, not a plastic one!)
➤ Think positive thoughts – 'breathe slowly', ' I can get through this', ' I'm not going to die!'
➤ If you are in a situation you really feel you can't handle, then try and get out of it for a short time. For instance, if you're in a long queue at the supermarket check out, ask the assistant to look after your trolley, and go outside for five minutes of fresh air. Or if you're driving, pull over to the side of the road.

➤ Don't worry about what other people are thinking. It really doesn't matter!

Prevention.
➤ Cut down on coffee, tea and alcohol, which can make you more excitable. The nicotine in cigarettes can have the same effect, so cut down on those too, or better still, stop altogether.
➤ Learn some relaxation techniques, and practise deep breathing.
➤ Try and identify situations that trigger attacks, then take action to make them less threatening. Just knowing you have an easy exit route can make a dramatic difference to your ability to cope. So, for instance, use an end check out at the supermarket, and an end of row seat at the cinema.
➤ Take general steps to reduce your stress levels if you can (see page 161).

Help from your doctor
➤ Your doctor may be able to refer you to a clinical psychologist who could help you face your fears using psychotherapy or teach you how to cope with them through gradual exposure to frightening and threatening situations.
➤ Counselling can help you to cope and deal with situations that cause anxiety, even if they seem to be outside your own control – such as housing or money worries.
➤ Tranquillizers can be helpful for relieving severe panic attacks. However, they are very addictive and should never be used for more than a few days at a time.

PELVIC INFLAMMATORY DISEASE

Pelvic inflammatory disease (often known as PID) means inflammation and infection of the reproductive organs – the womb, the Fallopian tubes and the ovaries.

In many cases it's caused by an infection spreading up from the vagina and cervix. The organisms responsible (either on their own, or as a mixture) include chlamydia, gonorrhoea and a group of bugs known as anaerobes. Sometimes these organisms produce a vaginal discharge, but in many cases there are no obvious symptoms of the initial infection until the signs of PID appear. Women with an IUCD or coil are more at risk of PID following a vaginal infection. PID can also occur after an abortion or miscarriage, and after childbirth.

Symptoms vary according to the severity of the infection and subsequent inflammation. They include:

➤ pelvic pain. This varies from a dull ache, to severe agonizing pain. The pain is often felt in the back, as well as deep in the pelvis. It may come and go, or it may be there all the time
➤ pain on intercourse, especially deep penetration. It may make having intercourse impossible
➤ heavy, painful periods
➤ bleeding in-between periods
➤ there may be a vaginal discharge, but in many cases severe PID occurs with no obvious discharge at all
➤ in more severe cases, women have a high temperature and feel very unwell.

Any woman with any of these symptoms should see a doctor as soon as possible. A skilled GP can make a fairly accurate diagnosis by giving the woman a thorough pelvic examination. This needs to be done with two hands (one in the vagina, one on the lower tummy wall). There is usually severe pain when the doctor touches, or moves the neck of, the womb. Beware of any doctor that makes the diagnosis just by feeling the tummy alone without doing an internal examination.

Further tests are not usually needed in the first instance, but an ultrasound scan can reveal characteristic swollen Fallopian tubes, and fluid in the pelvic space behind the womb. A laparoscopy is needed for an absolutely definitive diagnosis – but this is usually only done when symptoms persist for months despite treatment.

Treatment is with antibiotics. Although a vaginal swab may reveal the bug responsible for the infection, in many cases it's not possible to identify the exact cause. Often a mixture of bacteria are to blame, which can only be effectively treated using at least two different antibiotics for at least two weeks.

In the majority of cases, PID is a sexually transmitted disease, so it's important that the partners of all women affected have a check-up and treatment, even if there are no symptoms. This can prevent reinfection occurring. It's best not to have sex while you are having treatment – it tends to make the pain worse anyway.

PID is an important illness for women because it can cause scarring, and sometimes complete blockage, of the Fallopian tubes. It's a common cause of infertility. The tubal damage can also increase the risk of an ectopic pregnancy.

In some women it's also a cause of chronic, recurring pelvic pain. Repeated bouts of inflammation and pain occur which each require treatment with high dose antibiotics. Sometimes these attacks are triggered by having sex, sometimes they occur spontaneously.

Sometimes, recurrent bouts of pain are due to adhesions between the pelvic organs, which can be surgically divided using a laparoscope. In more severe cases, the only way to finally cure the pain is to remove the affected organs – either just the Fallopian tubes, or sometimes the womb and ovaries as well. Although this sounds drastic, it can give welcome relief for women who have suffered years of misery.

Prevention

PID can usually be prevented by:

➤ avoiding promiscuity. The more sexual partners you have, the greater the risk of catching a sexually transmitted disease

➤ using barrier contraception at all times, but especially when you have a new partner, or if you are worried that your partner is not being faithful to you

➤ getting prompt treatment at the first sign of a vaginal infection.

PELVIC PAIN

Pelvic pain is a common condition in women of all ages, and although it's often caused by a gynaecological problem, a bowel or urinary disorder may be to blame.

Apart from straightforward period pains, the most common gynaecological causes of pelvic pain are pelvic inflammatory disease (PID) and endometriosis (see page 62). Both can cause severe pain, but the pain of endometriosis tends to be much worse at period time, while the pain of acute PID is present all the time. Unlike endometriosis, PID can also cause a temperature and general feeling of malaise. Both can cause discomfort during sex, especially on deep penetration.

Chronic PID can also cause repeated bouts of less severe pain, which may be worse on one side of the pelvis than the other. The list of other causes includes ovarian cysts and fibroids (though these tend to cause discomfort rather than acute pain), irritable bowel syndrome (see page 116) and inflammation of the bladder.

If you suffer from pelvic pain it's important to see a doctor and to have it investigated. Sometimes the diagnosis can be made from a simple examination, but if you have persistent pain, a diagnostic laparoscopy (see page 118) may be required.

In some women even a laparoscopy does not reveal an obvious cause for recurrent bouts of pain. Unfortunately, some doctors then assume the pain is either due to irritable bowel syndrome, or 'all in the mind'. However, it now appears that enlarged pelvic veins may cause pain in many women who have apparently normal pelvic organs. This is known as pelvic congestion. It causes a pain that's worse on one side than the other, that tends to be present all the time as a dull ache, then flare up at certain times, especially after sex, or after standing up for a long time. Emotional stress seems to make the pain worse. A special pelvic X-ray using contrast dye may reveal the dilated veins, and give a firm diagnosis, but unfortunately this is only done in specialist centres. Treatment is with continuous progesterone tablets for several months, together in some cases with anti-depressants. All women with suspected pelvic congestion should have a trial of treatment, as it can be very successful.

PERIODS

Periods, (or to give them their proper medical term, menstruation) are due to the periodic shedding of the womb lining, together with a small amount of fresh blood. In most women it's an event that occurs approximately once a month – although anything from twenty-five to thirty-five days between the start of each period is quite normal.

Menstruation is controlled by a complicated cycle of change in the levels of the hormones oestrogen and progesterone, which are produced by the ovaries.

After each period there's an increase in the amount of oestrogen produced, which leads to a steady build up in the womb lining. After ovulation, (the release of an egg from one of the ovaries), there's initially a build up in the progesterone level. This alters the womb lining, preparing it for a pregnancy. If the egg isn't fertilized, there's a fall in the progesterone level, leading to shedding of the womb lining once the level goes below a threshold value – usually two weeks after ovulation.

Periods usually start around the age of eleven to twelve, although anything from ten to sixteen is regarded as normal. Periods continue up until the menopause, around the age of fifty. These years are the fertile time of a woman's life.

A normal period lasts for about five days, and on average, about 60ml of blood is lost – that's twelve teaspoonfuls. Any pain that occurs is usually worst on the first two days, while the heaviest blood flow is usually on the second and third days. It's normal to lose small clots, or small pieces of lining tissue, but the frequent passage of large clots or lumps is not normal.

Although periods can be a nuisance, many women have no trouble with them at all, but they do commonly cause problems, including pain or heavy, prolonged or erratic bleeding.

PERIOD PAINS

Pain is the most common problem caused by periods. It's a very distinct type of pain, which varies between a dull ache in the lower tummy to severe cramps. Often the pain spreads down the back, and can be felt in the front of the legs too.

Period pains (the proper medical term is dysmenorrhoea) can start at any time in a woman's reproductive life, but they are particularly common, and severe, when periods first begin, in the teenage years. The pain tends to ease off with increasing age, and often disappears completely after having a baby. The middle years (the twenties and thirties) are often pain-free for many women, but then pain may reoccur in the forties.

Period pains are linked with the production of the hormone prostoglandin, which causes the womb muscle to contract. It's also thought to be linked with the nausea, vomiting and occasional diarrhoea that some women experience at the beginning of each period. Women who suffer severe pains are thought to have high levels of prostaglandins.

In young women, pain may also be increased by a very tight cervix. In most cases, especially in younger women, there's no obvious cause for the pain, and apart from the fact that they can wreck your life for two days each month, they are nothing to worry about. Occasionally, however, there can be an underlying cause. In particular, period pains that suddenly become more severe, when they have previously been very mild, should always be investigated.

Any pelvic infection, or PID, can cause more painful, and heavier periods than before (see page 134). Endometriosis (see page 62) can also cause period pains that start a few days before each period, building to a peak of very severe pain on the first or second day of bleeding.

Fibroids can also be to blame, and are a common cause for pains reoccurring in older women. Copper-containing coils such as the Multiload, and the Gynae-T can also cause quite severe pains, especially in women who have not had children.

Self-help

➤ Painkillers available from the chemist ease mild pains. Drugs that reduce prostoglandin levels, particularly ibuprofen, are more effective than ordinary paracetamol. Codeine is stronger still, and combined with aspirin is a good remedy for period pains.

➤ A hot bath can be very relaxing and help to ease cramps. Try adding a few drops of either chamomile or sweet marjoram essential oil. Alternatively, ask a friend to gently massage your back and lower abdomen with a few drops of these oils added to either a carrier oil or lotion.

➤ Getting uptight can make period pains worse. Practise relaxation exercises in between periods, then put them into good use when the pain strikes.

➤ Some women find that exercise helps too. A brisk walk or a swim may help to take your mind off the pain.

➤ Some women find that a daily supplement of gammolenic acid in the form of starflower or evening primrose oil is helpful.

Help from your doctor
Many women seem concerned that it's wasting time to go to a doctor with period pains. This is rubbish. It's a genuine problem, and there's a lot that can be done to help. For straightforward pains in young women a pelvic examination is rarely needed, unless there are other symptoms as well. But all women with sudden, more severe pain or other symptoms, such as pain during intercourse, should have the cause investigated, and this should include a pelvic examination.

Medical treatments
➤ Stronger and more effective anti-prostaglandins, such as mefenamic acid, are available on prescription.

➤ Muscle relaxants, such as hyoscine, can ease cramps and can be taken in addition to other painkillers.

➤ Anti-sickness pills can help to relieve nausea.

➤ If these don't work, the combined oral contraceptive pill can have a dramatic effect at relieving period pains. It stops ovulation and the artificial withdrawal bleed that occurs in the pill-free week each month is usually much less painful, and lighter, than a normal period. If you're not keen to take the Pill all the time, you can take it for just a few months to ease period pains during an important time, for instance, during exams, or starting a new job.

➤ In very severe cases, widening the cervix under anaesthetic may help, but this is rarely done nowadays.

HEAVY PERIODS
It's often difficult to judge whether you have heavy periods or not.

What seems heavy for one woman may be light for another. Unless you weigh your sanitary towels, it can be impossible to know accurately if you are losing more than the average 60ml each month.

A good indicator can be the pattern of sanitary towel use. If you need to change a super tampon, or towel, at least once an hour, if you have to wear two pads at once, or if you pass large clots, then your periods are heavier than normal. This also applies if your periods last more than a week, with heavy flow for more than four days.

Although they may seem nothing more than a nuisance, heavy periods shouldn't be ignored. Apart from the additional cost burden of all those sanitary towels, the excess blood lost is a common cause of iron-deficiency anaemia in women. Heavy periods can also be the first indicator of a gynaecological problem.

It's normal for periods to become slightly heavier with increasing age, particularly after having a baby. With each pregnancy, the womb enlarges slightly (it only goes back completely to its pre-pregnancy size after the menopause), and fibroids develop in about a fifth of women, (see page 171). Although these are often completely harmless (they never turn cancerous), fibroids can grow to a large size and cause very heavy bleeding, particularly if they distort the lining of the womb.

Heavy periods can also be caused by a pelvic infection, and also by ordinary copper coils. They can also be due to polyps, which are small outgrowths, usually the size of a grape, from the womb lining.

Heavy, and often erratic periods, usually occur in slightly older women, in their late thirties and forties. Often there's no obvious cause at all, although some gynaecologists blame an upset in the cyclical secretion of the hormones oestrogen and progesterone.

P

Self-help
Anti-prostaglandin tablets, such as ibuprofen, taken regularly every four hours, may reduce blood flow slightly. However, all women with heavy periods should see a doctor for a check up.

Help from your doctor
All women with heavy periods should have a thorough pelvic examination. This can give an indication of the cause, such as fibroids or a pelvic infection. A vaginal ultrasound scan can usually confirm the size of fibroids and also reveal whether the womb lining is abnormally thickened, or whether there are polyps present.

Medical treatments

➤ The first treatment is usually hormone therapy. The combined contraceptive pill is very effective, but if this is not suitable, progesterone tablets, taken for either one or two weeks before each period, can help to reduce the flow, and control an erratic cycle.

➤ Tablets that close down tiny bleeding vessels, such as ethamsylate or tranexamic acid, are better still at reducing menstrual blood loss. They are taken four times a day, but only when the flow is heavy.

➤ The new Mirena IUCD thins the womb lining and is showing promise as a very effective treatment for heavy periods, especially when there is no obvious cause (see page 74).

Surgical treatments

Surgery may be needed if other treatments fail to control bleeding. Surgery may also be the most appropriate treatment in some cases, such as large fibroids.

➤ In the past, a D and C (see page 51) was often performed for heavy periods, but this operation is becoming increasing obsolete. Unless a polyp is present (and removed) it just doesn't work!

➤ The newer version of the D and C is a hysteroscopy, where the womb cavity is viewed through a special telescope. Under anaesthetic, this is passed up into the womb via the cervix. It's far more accurate than a D and C, and allows the gynaecologist to remove tiny polyps that might otherwise be missed.

➤ In cases where there is no obvious cause for heavy periods, it may help to remove the whole of the womb lining, using either hot cautery or a laser. Although this operation, known as endometrial ablation, can be very successful, it does not always stop periods altogether, and some women do suffer increased period pains afterwards. In some cases, heavy periods return and later surgery is needed. Women considering this option should always discuss the risks fully beforehand, and make sure that the gynaecologist concerned is fully trained in the technique (see Useful Addresses).

➤ Isolated fibroids can sometimes be removed from the womb (a myomectomy). This operation is usually reserved for women who have not yet completed their families and wish to retain their fertility.

➤ If periods are very heavy, especially if there are several fibroids present, the best solution is often to have a hysterectomy (see page 100). This may sound drastic, but there are many women who will testify that having their womb removed gave them a new lease of life!

ERRATIC PERIODS

Many women do not have regular monthly periods. Irregular periods, which occur in a completely unpredictable fashion, are usually linked to erratic ovulation. In some cases, occasional erratic periods occur when the hormone cycle is in disarray and there has been no ovulation at all. Erratic ovulation and irregular periods are particularly common at the two extremes of reproductive life – that is, for the first few years when periods first begin, and for the few years leading up to the menopause. Erratic periods are normal when weaning a child from the breast. Another common cause is progesterone based contraceptives, such as the progesterone-only pill, and the rod system Norplant, which can cause erratic ovulation.

Some women always have erratic ovulation and erratic periods, for no obvious reason. This is nothing to worry about and requires no treatment unless unpredictable bleeding is a problem, in which case the most effective treatment is to go on the combined contraceptive pill. The only other time that treatment is indicated is if the erratic ovulation is causing fertility problems. This is the only time when it is appropriate to use drugs such as clomiphene, which stimulate ovulation.

In some women erratic ovulation is due to polycystic ovaries, which happens when tiny cysts form in the ovaries and there is an imbalance in the hormones FSH and LH, which stimulate the ovaries (see page 144). If the only symptom is erratic periods then no treatment is required. However, if there are other symptoms, such as acne and excessive body hair, treatment with the contraceptive pill Dianette can be of benefit. It can improve the skin, and give regular bleeds.

Erratic, infrequent periods can also be caused by excessive weight loss, and excessive exercise. Occasional periods can also be due to hormonal problems, such as an overactive thyroid gland or an excess of the hormone prolactin. Any change in your menstrual cycle for no obvious reason, should always be investigated by a doctor.

BLEEDING IN-BETWEEN PERIODS

The only time that vaginal bleeding should occur is during a period. Bleeding at other times is not normal, and although it's rarely due to a serious cause, it should always be investigated by a doctor.

Common causes include:

➤ the combined pill. Occasional 'breakthrough bleeding' is quite common, but if it occurs repeatedly several months in a row, then

it's an indication that a change of formulation, with a different balance of hormones is needed
➤ a cervical erosion (see page 37). This can cause bleeding particularly after intercourse
➤ a cervical polyp. Again, this tends to cause bleeding after intercourse
➤ in older women, a dry, inflamed vagina is due to lack of oestrogen. This should only cause slight red/brown spotting, and not bright red blood loss.

More seriously, bleeding in between periods can be due to:
➤ pelvic inflammatory disease (PID)
➤ cancer of the cervix, the womb, or the ovary. In older women especially, bleeding that occurs after the menopause needs urgent attention.

PILES (OR HAEMORRHOIDS)

These are swollen veins just inside or outside the opening of the anus. They are common in women, especially during pregnancy and after childbirth. They are also more common in people who have a tendency to constipation and strain to open their bowels. The tendency to develop piles can also run in families. Symptoms include itching and discomfort, lumpiness around the anus, and fresh bleeding. This usually occurs during and after passing a motion.

Self-help
Rectal bleeding should always be investigated by a doctor – never assume it's 'just piles'.
    Symptoms of piles can be eased by:
➤ avoiding constipation. Eat a high-fibre diet, with added bran
➤ not straining on the toilet. Try to avoid spending ages on the loo (read your favourite book somewhere else!)
➤ creams such as Anusol (available from chemists) can ease itching and discomfort. Suppositories are more effective for piles inside the anus.

Help from your doctor
Persistently troublesome piles can be treated with an injection of phenol, which blocks the vein concerned. Alternatively, piles can be surgically tied, or removed.

POLYCYSTIC OVARIES (PCO)

PCO syndrome can cause several symptoms, including erratic, infrequent periods, excess body hair, a greasy skin, and obesity. It is also a well-recognised cause of infertility, although many women with PCO do manage to conceive without too much difficulty.

The condition can be diagnosed by testing blood hormone levels, together with an ovarian ultrasound scan. If levels of the hormones LH (from the pituitary gland) and testosterone (from the ovaries) are high, and numerous tiny cysts can be seen in the ovaries on the ultrasound then the diagnosis is PCO.

Treatment depends on the symptoms, and whether a pregnancy is desired. The drug cyproterone acetate reduces testosterone levels, and helps greasy skin, acne, and excess body hair. It's usually given in the form of the contraceptive pill Dianette, which also has the benefit of allowing regular withdrawal bleeds. For women who are trying to conceive, drugs that stimulate ovulation, such as Clomiphene or Pergonal, are used. In some cases, surgically removing a wedge-shaped piece of ovarian tissue may be helpful (although this operation has rather gone out of fashion in recent years).

PRE-MENSTRUAL SYNDROME (PMS)

It's rare to find a woman who has never noticed any change in her body, or her feelings, just before a period. Some women have only mild pre-menstrual symptoms, which they can mostly ignore. Some have good months and bad months. Others find they suffer dreadfully and consistently, for up to two weeks every single month.

There are reckoned to be more than 150 symptoms associated with PMS, so it's impossible to list them all. They can be divided into two groups – mental problems and physical symptoms. Mental problems include tension (PMT), depression, aggression, anxiety, tiredness, poor concentration, food cravings and a change (usually a decrease) in libido. Common physical symptoms include headaches, sore, tender breasts and a bloated tummy.

No one is sure of the exact cause of PMS, but a change in the ratio of the hormones oestrogen and progesterone is thought to be to blame. Progesterone levels rise in the week following ovulation (seven to fourteen days before a period) but in the final seven days before bleeding occurs, levels plummet along with a less dramatic fall in oestrogen levels.

Self-help for PMS

➤ First of all, make sure that you really are suffering from PMS. Keep a daily dairy of your symptoms and when your period occurs. Be honest. PMS symptoms only occur in the two weeks before each period. If you are getting symptoms at other times, you can't blame PMS, and more importantly, PMS treatments probably won't help you.

➤ Check your diet. Tension, tiredness and mood swings can often be eased by stabilizing your blood sugar level. Eat regularly, at least once every three hours. Don't skip meals. Concentrate on foods that will give long-lasting energy, such as wholemeal bread and crackers, and pasta. Even if you crave chocolate and sweets avoid them if possible, as they can cause wild swings in blood sugar levels, first high, then low.

➤ If you're prone to bloating, cut down on salt, especially in the two weeks before each period. This means avoiding table salt, salty foods such as smoked fish and meats, and salted crisps and nuts.

➤ Caffeine, particularly in large amounts, can cause irritability. Switch to decaffeinated coffee, tea and cola. Better still, cut these out altogether and replace with water, fruit juice and herbal teas. Cut down slowly however, especially if you're used to drinking large amounts of ordinary coffee, as sudden caffeine withdrawal can cause a thumping headache.

➤ Vitamin B6, or pyridoxine, can ease many PMS symptoms. The dose is 50mg daily, throughout your cycle. Don't take more than this – it can be dangerous. It's available directly from chemists, and also on prescription from GPs.

➤ Gammolenic acid is another good all-round remedy, and it is particularly effective at reducing breast tenderness. Aim to take 500mg daily. It's found in evening primrose oil and starflower oil. Some GPs will prescribe evening primrose oil for severe cyclical breast pain.

➤ The anti-prostoglandin ibuprofen is a good remedy for pre-menstrual aches and pains.

➤ Avoid excess stress if possible during the pre-menstrual weeks. Make sure you get plenty of sleep, and allow yourself some daily relaxation time. Getting wound up and overtired only makes PMS worse. To encourage relaxation, try adding a couple of drops of either lavender or rose oil to your bath each night. Or ask a good friend to give you a soothing massage, with lavender or rose oil added to either a carrier oil or lotion.

Help from your doctor

Although there are several drug treatments available that can really help PMS, there's no single one that's universally successful. A drug that's a miracle cure for one woman may not help another. So it's really a case of 'try it and see' until you find a treatment that works for you. But don't chop and change too quickly – give each treatment at least a three month trial.

Most hormonal treatments work by dampening down the fluctuating levels of the hormones oestrogen and progesterone. Effective drugs available include:

➤ the combined contraceptive pill. This is especially suitable for younger women who also need effective contraception. Preparations that contain differing levels of hormones (particularly 'tri-phasic' pills), are best avoided, as these cause PMS in some women

➤ progestogens. These include the progesterone-only pill (taken all the time) or better still, natural progesterone suppositories, used only in the two weeks before each period. If you don't fancy suppositories, dydrogesterone tablets, again taken for only two weeks each month, are effective for some women

➤ danazol – higher doses often stop periods altogether, but a special low-dose formulation is available as a treatment for PMS

➤ in severe cases, Gnrh analogues, such as buserilin, can be used (see page 64). These switch the ovaries off altogether, and though they can be very effective against PMS they can cause menopausal-type symptoms. Because of this, they should not be used on a long-term basis

➤ in older women, hormone-replacement therapy (HRT), particularly in the form of skin patches, can ease PMS.

Diuretic pills, which help the body get rid of excess water, can ease pre-menstrual bloating. They should only be taken just before each period, and not all the time.

When pre-menstrual depression is severe, a course of anti-depressant tablets can be very helpful. In these cases the drugs should be taken all the time, for at least three months. However, unlike tranquillizers, they are not addictive.

PROLAPSE

A prolapse is a change, usually downwards or outwards, in the normal position of one of the body organs. Although the term can be used for a slipped disc in the back, it's more commonly used when the womb drops from its normal position, down into the vagina. It's caused by stretching and weakening of the ligaments that support the womb, usually as a result of pregnancy and childbirth. It's a condition that tends to occur more often, and more severely, in women who have had several children, and who are overweight.

In mild cases, there may be no symptoms at all, but as the womb drops further into the vagina, many women are aware of 'something coming down'. In severe cases, the neck of the womb, or cervix, may be visible outside the entrance to the vagina. The vaginal walls often prolapse too. The most common part affected is the front wall, when the bladder bulges into the vagina (a cystocele). This can cause stress incontinence. If the back wall is weakened, the rectum can bulge into the vagina (a rectocele). Both these conditions can occur without any prolapse of the womb.

Self-help
➤ Pelvic floor exercises (see page 103) can help to strengthen the muscles of the vagina, and can help to both prevent and improve a prolapse. These exercises should be routine for all new mums, for at least three months after the baby is born!
➤ Losing weight can help to ease pressure on the womb.
➤ Smoking, and the coughing that goes with it, can make a prolapse worse. Yet another reason to stop as soon as possible!
➤ Regular exercise will also help to maintain muscle tone and reduce the risk of a prolapse occuring.

Help from your doctor
All types of prolapse can be treated surgically. The vaginal walls can be tightened and strengthened – a repair operation. This is usually done from below, and only requires a few days in hospital. Gynaecologists usually only do this type of operation on women who have completed their families – having another baby can undo all their good work!

The best treatment for a prolapsed womb is to remove it, and unless it is enlarged as well, this too can be done via the vagina (a vaginal hysterectomy – see page 100).

For women who do not want an operation (or, as may be the case in elderly women, are not fit enough for surgery), a special plastic ring pessary can be inserted into the vagina, to hold the womb in place, and prevent it from dropping further. These pessaries need changing every three months, but this can usually be done by a GP

PSORIASIS

This is a skin condition that causes patches of thick, itchy, white-silvery scales. It can occur on any part of the body, but the front of the knees, the backs of the elbows, the front of the shins, and the scalp are the areas most often affected. It's caused by the cells of the skin turning over up to ten times faster than normal. Often there's no obvious reason for this, but in some people psoriasis tends to appear at times of emotional or physical stress. It can also have a tendency to run in families.

Self-help
➤ Prevent dry skin generally by a regular daily application of moisturizing cream or lotion all over, and especially in areas that tend to be affected.
➤ Creams containing coal tar can help to slow down the rapid cell turn over.
➤ Psoriasis often improves on exposure to sunlight.
➤ If possible avoid becoming overtired or stressed.

Help from your doctor
➤ Creams and lotions containing calcipotriol are often very effective.
➤ Alternatively, dithranol cream can be used, but it can be irritating and stains clothing.
➤ Steroid creams do usually clear psoriasis, but once stopped the lesions often recur and are worse than before.
➤ Severe lesions can be treated in hospitals by a special form of light therapy known as PUVA.

PUBERTY

This is the time when the sexual maturity begins. In girls, it usually begins between the ages of ten and twelve, a couple of years earlier than boys, but any time between ten and sixteen is normal. The first sign is usually breast development, followed by the appearance of pubic hair. The first period is usually about a year later than this – the average age in the UK is now twelve and a half. By then pubic and underarm hair are well established.

Occasionally, puberty can start at an extremely young age, due to abnormal hormone secretion. More common is delayed puberty, due to low hormone levels. Although this may occur for no obvious reason, excessive physical exercise, or an extremely low body weight, may be to blame.

R

RAYNAUD'S DISEASE

In this condition, the small arteries supplying blood to the fingers and toes go into spasm in cold temperatures. This causes extreme pain, as the fingers turn first white, then blue. When the circulation returns, they throb and turn red. It particularly affects young women.

Treatment is mainly preventative, by keeping fingers and toes as warm as possible in cold weather. This means wearing thick mittens (which are warmer than gloves) and warm, woollen socks. Sufferers should avoid wearing tight shoes which can lower the circulation to toes – boots that allow space for the toes to wriggle are best. Special electrically heated mittens (driven by a battery) are available for those who are severely affected. Smoking, which narrows blood vessels, makes the condition worse. If necessary, drugs that widen the blood vessels, such as nifedipine, may be helpful. Ginkobiloba (extracted from the Sinko tree), available from all chemists, has been shown to improve circulation and reduce symptoms in some patients. Make sure the product you buy is high in active glycosides.

REPETITIVE STRAIN INJURY (RSI)

Any ligament or tendon can become inflamed with persistent use, causing pain and stiffness. Women in certain professions are at increased risk, particularly typists and keyboard operators (when inflammation can affect the finger, thumb and wrist joints), hairdressers (hands, wrists and elbows) and cleaners (again, hands and arms).

The best treatment is to completely rest the affected joint until the inflammation subsides. This may take several weeks. Anti-inflammatory drugs can speed up this process, often by simply applying a cream three times a day.

RSI can often be prevented by taking regular breaks from repetitive work, at least once every two hours. Keyboard operators should also make sure that their desk, chair, screen and keyboard are in the best position to avoid any unnecessary strain on any joint. Advice on this can usually be obtained from the company health and safety officer.

RHEUMATOID ARTHRITIS
(see Arthritis page 19.)

RHESUS FACTOR

The rhesus system is based on either the presence, or absence, of antigens, known as rhesus factors, in blood. 85 percent of people have blood containing the Rhesus D antigen, and are therefore Rhesus positive. The remaining 15 percent, who don't have the factor, are rhesus negative. The rhesus system is completely separate from the ABO system (the usual blood grouping test) that determines a person's blood group.

Problems can arise if a rhesus negative woman bears a baby who is rhesus positive (which can happen if the baby's father is rhesus positive). The rhesus factor can spill over from the baby into the mother, usually at the time of birth, who then forms antibodies against it. In subsequent pregnancies, these rhesus antibodies can destroy the red blood cells in the unborn baby, causing severe anaemia, and sometimes the death of the baby.

All women who are rhesus negative should be given a special injection, called Anti-D, immediately after they have given birth. This mops up, and destroys any rhesus positive cells from the baby before the mother has a chance to react to them. This also applies to rhesus negative women who have a miscarriage or termination. The risk of rhesus disease only occurs in rhesus negative women with a rhesus positive baby. If both parents are rhesus negative, then the baby will be rhesus negative.

ROSACEA

This is a skin disorder affecting the face, usually across the nose and cheeks. Pustules appear, resembling acne, and there is redness and flushing, which is often most noticeable after hot drinks, alcohol or spicy food. In most cases, the cause isn't known, but it can be due to overuse of strong steroid creams on the face. It's most common in middle-aged women, who often mistake it for acne.

Treatment is either with tetracycline antibiotics (taken by mouth), or Metronidazole gel (applied on the affected areas). Treatment usually has to be continued for months, or even years.

RUBELLA (OR GERMAN MEASLES)

In itself, German measles is a relatively minor illness. The virus can, however, have devastating effects on an unborn baby. Symptoms include a slight fever and swollen glands, together with a faint red rash that starts on the face and spreads downwards. In adults, particularly, the joints may ache and swell, but overall symptoms rarely last for more than a few days.

The infection can be confirmed by blood tests. All women should make sure that they are immune to the illness, and certainly before they stop using contraception in order to conceive. All women who are not immune should be vaccinated.

Unborn babies in the first four months of pregnancy are most at risk from the infection, which can cause deafness, heart disease, mental retardation and cataracts.

R

S

SEASONAL AFFECTIVE DISORDER (SAD)

This is a recurrent form of depression that occurs every winter. Its severity varies, but up to as many as one in five people are thought to be affected to some degree. It's far more common in women than men. Symptoms include tiredness, excessive sleepiness, irritability, poor concentration, and a change in eating habits, often with a craving for sweet foods. Symptoms usually start as the days become noticeably shorter in the autumn, and then improve as the days lengthen again in the spring.

The exact cause isn't known, but the increased hours of darkness during the winter may lead to an increase in the levels of the hormone melatonin, which is produced by the pineal gland, a tiny pea-sized structure in the brain.

Self-help
➤ Get outside as much as possible during the winter, to make the most of what little daylight there is.
➤ To increase your general sense of well-being, eat a well-balanced diet, and take plenty of exercise.

Help from your doctor
➤ Some patients benefit from anti-depressants, particularly the newer SSRI types (such as Fluoxetine and Paroxetine). Treatment is only required during the winter, and the tablets can be stopped without difficulty in the spring.
➤ Light therapy can be very helpful for those severely affected. This involves sitting in front of a special powerful light box for several hours each day. These boxes emit light that is up to twenty times stronger than normal indoor lighting. Unfortunately, light treatment is rarely available on the NHS.

SEXUAL PROBLEMS

These can be divided into two groups. Firstly, a lack of sex drive, or low libido; and secondly, problems enjoying sex to the full when it occurs. Many women suffer from one or either of these, a few from both.

LOW LIBIDO

A woman's desire for sex is affected by both physical and emotional health. It's perfectly normal to have times when, even if you are in a loving and satisfactory relationship, you don't feel like sex. The ups and downs of normal everyday living can inevitably affect your sex life. Feeling over-tired or stressed, or even a minor squabble can turn off your libido.

The changing levels of hormones that occur in each menstrual cycle can also naturally affect the sex drive. At the time of ovulation, when oestrogen levels peak, many women experience a upward surge in their sex drive. But following ovulation, as progesterone levels rise, libido normally falls.

Before the menopause, the ovaries also produce a small amount of the male hormone testosterone, and this is thought to have a positive effect on a woman's libido. After the menopause, the levels of both oestrogen and testosterone fall dramatically, and this in turn can cause a marked decrease in the sex drive.

After childbirth, sheer exhaustion means that many new mums don't feel like sex. But breast-feeding mums, in addition, have high levels of the hormone prolactin, and this can also reduce the sex drive.

Some drugs, particularly some blood pressure treatments, sedatives and also some combined contraceptives can also lower libido. Any physical illness, including a nasty dose of the 'flu or a heavy cold, as well as more serious conditions, can also affect the sex drive. Low libido is also common in depression. If sex is painful, or has been in the past, it can also, not surprisingly, reduce the desire to try it again.

However, the sex drive is far more commonly affected by relationship problems. Low libido can be one of the first signs that you are dissatisfied with other aspects of your life together. In some cases it may be a signal that it's time for the relationship to end – in others, it's a sign that the your relationship together needs some attention. Lack of libido can also be sign of boredom. At the start of a new relationship, most couples have a very active sex life, and it's quite normal for sex to become a little less frequent as time passes. But if it gets to the stage when it's dull and routine, it can be a big turn-off.

S

Self-help

➤ Try and work out why you don't feel like sex. Is it because you really don't love your partner any more, and you don't want to be intimate? Or are you happy to have cuddles, but don't want to have sex?

➤ If you think your relationship may be to blame, then don't sit back and do nothing. Talk to your partner, and try and work out some positive steps to improve matters.

➤ If boredom has crept in and you can't spice things up on your own, try either hiring a sexual instruction video, or a book.

If it's not your relationship

➤ Avoid becoming overtired. Make sure you have time with your partner when you're not exhausted.

➤ Take positive steps to reduce your stress levels (see page 161).

➤ Don't expect too much if you've just had a baby, or a physical illness. Give your body time to recover.

➤ If sex hurts, see below.

Help from your doctor

➤ Counselling can help if you are unable to solve your relationship problems on your own. You can either arrange this via your GP, or alternatively, contact your local branch of Relate.

➤ Check with your doctor if any pills or medications you are taking (including contraceptives) may be affecting your sex drive. If so, change to a different formulation.

➤ Hormone-replacement therapy (HRT) can often boost sex drive in older women. If standard HRT, in normal doses is insufficient, then adding a small dose of testosterone may be helpful. This is usually given via a small implant inserted deep under the skin of either the lower abdomen or the buttocks.

➤ Specialist psycho-sexual counselling can usually help when there is no obvious cause for a low sex drive. It can teach you techniques so you can learn to focus on your needs, and learn to enjoy sex again.

PAINFUL SEX

There are two distinct areas where sex can hurt – either in and around the entrance to the vagina at the start of penetration; or deep inside the pelvis, which is usually felt more during intense thrusting.

Vaginal pain can be caused by:
➤ dryness and lack of lubrication, which means that the penis chafes, rather than glides inside the vagina. This can be due to lack of foreplay, but in older women may be due to low oestrogen levels
➤ vaginal inflammation, due to either an allergy, or an infection
➤ a tight vagina. This is more common when you first start having sex, and also after childbirth, if stitches have been required. But it can also be the sign of a deeper emotional problem, or worry, about having sex.

Deep pelvic pain on intercourse can be due to:
➤ your partner thrusting too deep, and hitting your cervix. Try changing your position, and ask your partner to be a bit gentler
➤ pelvic inflammatory disease (see page 134). This is more likely if you've had a vaginal discharge, heavier or more painful periods than normal, or bleeding in-between periods
➤ endometriosis (see page 62)
More rarely, deep pain during intercourse can be due to an ovarian cyst, fibroids, or adhesions from previous infections or surgery, or an inflamed bowel.

Self-help
➤ Make sure you are fully aroused and well-lubricated before you try and have penetrative sex. This means allowing adequate time for foreplay. In addition, try smearing a layer of lubricating jelly, such as K-Y, on your partner's penis before he tries to enter you.
➤ If your vagina is dry and itchy, stop using bubble baths and perfumed soaps, and never douche.
➤ If you have a thick, itchy discharge and a sore vagina, you may have thrush (see page 164). Treatment for this is available directly from chemists.
➤ If you tense up before penetration, take things very slowly, and give yourself plenty of time to relax beforehand. Don't feel compelled to have intercourse every time you're with your partner. It may help if he gently widens the vaginal entrance with his fingers before he tries to enter with his penis.

Help from your doctor
➤ Deep pain on intercourse should always be investigated and treated by a doctor as soon as possible.

➤ The hormone oestrogen can help to ease a dry, uncomfortable vagina in older women. It can either be given in the form of conventional HRT, or as a cream that's applied to the vagina and surrounding area.

➤ Persistent vaginal soreness, or a discharge, should also be investigated and treated by your doctor.

➤ Persistent vaginal tightness following childbirth can often be eased by using special vaginal dilators (small plastic cones).

➤ Tightness due to psychological reasons can often be helped by specialist psycho-sexual counselling, or sex therapy.

SEXUALLY TRANSMITTED DISEASES (STDs)

A large number of infections can be passed on during close sexual contact. Some, such as herpes (see page 95), warts (see page 186) scabies and pubic lice, can be transmitted by close body contact alone. Others, such as gonorrhoea (see page 86) trichomonas (see page 169) and chlamydia (see page 41) are more usually transmitted during full penetrative intercourse. Syphilis also still occurs, but is more common in the homosexual community.

Most STDs, once correctly diagnosed, can be successfully treated. However, there is no cure as yet for either Hepatits B and HIV (see page 10), both of which can be passed on via contaminated needles as well as by unprotected sex.

You can reduce your risk of catching an STD by

➤ avoiding promiscuity. The greater the number of sexual partners that you have, the greater the risk

➤ using barrier contraceptives, particularly condoms (male or female). These can both be used in addition to a hormonal method, such as the Pill, if you wish.

If you are worried that you may have a STD, then see a doctor straight away. The best place to go for a prompt diagnosis and treatment is your local hospital department of Genito-Urinary Medicine. You do not need a referral letter from your GP, and your visit there will be completely confidential.

SKIN CARE

Your skin plays a major part in your appearance and attractiveness. It can also be a good indicator of general health and well-being.

The cells that make up the outer layer of skin (or epidermis) are continuously turning over, with new cells being produced at the

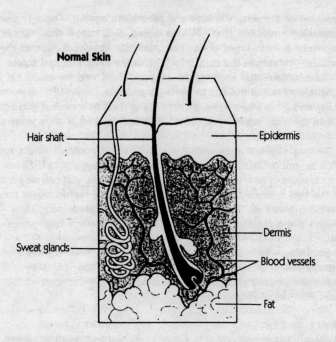

Normal Skin

Hair shaft

Epidermis

Dermis

Sweat glands

Blood vessels

Fat

bottom as dead cells are shed at the top. In young women it takes about a month for the skin to completely 'renew' itself, but this process slows down with increasing age, and this can result in slightly duller, thickened skin. The deeper layer of skin (or dermis) contains collagen and elastin, two proteins that give skin strength and make it supple. These are also affected by age, becoming thinner and less strong.

As with the rest of the body, a balanced diet, regular exercise and plenty of rest and sleep are vital for good skin. Avoiding smoking and excessive amounts of alcohol are important too. But by far and away the most damaging factor for skin is exposure to the ultraviolet rays in sunlight.

SUNLIGHT AND SUNSCREENS

There are two types of ultraviolet rays which damage skin, UVA and UVB. UVB rays only make up about 10 percent of the energy from the sun, but they are 1,000 times more damaging than UVA. They cause redness, burning and skin cancer. UVA rays can penetrate deeper into the skin and cause permanent damage, which is

S

revealed as dryness, wrinkles and premature ageing. There is also increasing evidence that UVA rays can also cause skin cancer. Exposure to both types of ray can stimulate the production of the pigment melanin in the skin, which gives the skin a tanned colour.

To maintain the appearance of your skin, and to avoid skin cancer, stay out of the sun as much as possible, especially between 11am and 2pm, when the sun's rays are at their strongest. If you are out in the sun, cover up as much as possible, and always wear a wide brimmed hat.

Protect exposed skin with a sunscreen that contains filters for UVA as well as UVB. The 'Sun Protection Factor' applies to UVB and is a measure of how many times longer than normal you can stay out in the sun without burning. For good skin, you should never use anything less than SPF 15. UVA protection is rated using stars – always use a product with three or four, which offers high protection.

Sunbeds, which usually emit UVA rays, are not much safer than natural strong sunlight. They don't cause burning, but they can cause premature ageing, and there is increasing evidence that they can cause skin cancer.

SKIN CANCER

There are three types of skin cancer – melanoma, basal cell carcinoma and squamous cell carcinoma. All three are becoming much more common, as tanning, and therefore high sun exposure, has become more fashionable.

The most dangerous by far is malignant melanoma. This can occur in people of all ages. About 50 percent of melanomas occur in a pre-existing mole. People who are fair skinned, with red or fair hair, blue eyes and freckles, and who tend to burn, rather than tan, and who have more than fifty moles are more at risk.

Watch out for a mole that:
➤ has an uneven colour, especially if it has recently changed and developed an irregular edge
➤ bleeds or itches
➤ is growing
➤ has a crusted top.

The sooner a melanoma is caught and treatment started, the greater the chance of a cure.

Daily care

Most skin only needs to be cleaned once a day. Water can actually dry the skin, and a quick shower is generally better for skin than a long soak in a hot bath. Most soaps are alkaline, and can disrupt the skin's normally slightly acidic secretions, leading to a dry, taut sensation. Special moisturising soaps or cleansing bars, which are less alkaline, are more suitable for women with very dry skin. All skins, apart from those that are very oily, benefit from a dose of moisturiser, which is best applied when the skin is still slightly damp and warm. This should be a year-round routine for the whole body, not just the face!

Cost is not a necessarily a good indicator of quality. One of the best body moisturisers is aqueous cream, available very cheaply from chemists. This has the added benefit of being free from any perfumes that can irritate sensitive skin. Women with sensitive skin should take care to avoid biological washing powders, especially for underwear, or other clothes that fit closely to the skin, and to use unperfumed soap for washing.

It's possible to waste a large amount of money on face creams that claim to reduce lines and wrinkles. Many only have a temporary 'plumping out' effect, but those containing alpha hydroxy acids, (AHAs, or fruit acids) do appear to have a genuinely beneficial effect by speeding up the process of cell shedding and renewal. Creams containing the Vitamin A derivative tretinoin (Retinova, and retin A) can also help to smooth fine lines and wrinkles, and improve skin texture by strengthening the collagen fibres in the deep layer of the skin. Both of these are only available on prescription, and side effects, including excessive redness and irritation, are quite common.

It's important to choose a foundation that's suitable for your skin type. Women with dry skins should opt for an oil-based product – those with an oily skin, one that is water-based. Try and also choose a foundation that's free from added perfumes (to reduce the risk of allergy), non-comogenic (that is, won't clog pores and cause spots) and contains an added sunscreen.

S

SLIMMING PILLS

There are various different drugs which can be used to try and aid slimming. Many of them just don't work, while others are dangerous and addictive.

Water tablets, or diuretics
These make you pass more urine. They can be useful if you retain water before a period, but in other circumstances your body will readjust the balance as soon as you have something to drink. Even small doses can cause a dry mouth, and larger doses can cause dehydration.

Laxatives
These just empty out the waste matter from the bowel a little quicker than normal. Although your weight will go down dramatically by a pound or two, it will gradually creep up again over the next couple of days, as your bowel naturally refills.

Appetite suppressants
As their name suggests, these reduce your appetite so it is easier to diet. They are related to amphetamines, and can be addictive. For a short time they can make you feel happier than normal, but as the effect wears off, you can feel low and depressed. They can also have dangerous side effects, particularly for the heart.

Most GPs won't prescribe appetite suppressants at all, but they are available from private clinics. Anyone taking them should have a thorough medical check-up first, and treatment should be for a maximum of eight weeks.

Bulking agents
These are the safest of all the pills available to aid dieting. Most are based on methyl cellulose, a plant fibre which expands dramatically with water, and which isn't absorbed into the body. Taken with a glass of water before a meal, a couple of tablets can fill up the stomach, so that you eat less. Sadly, the effect wears off and many people find they feel hungry an hour or so later!

If you do obtain slimming pills from a private clinic, always make sure you know exactly what you are taking. The bottle should be clearly labelled with the name of the drug (not with just a number). Some less scrupulous clinics do hand out concoctions of pills (including thyroid hormones) that can be particularly dangerous if you have high blood pressure, a heart condition, or if you are involved in a serious accident.

SMOKING

Smoking is a major health hazard, causing approximately 100,000 deaths each year in the UK. An increasing number of women are being affected by smoking-related diseases. Smoking doesn't just cause lung cancer – it is also a major contributory factor to cancer of the cervix, mouth and throat, and to heart disease and narrowed arteries throughout the body.

It also cause chronic inflammation in the lungs, leading to permanent shortness of breath, and persistent wheezing and coughing.

In women, smoking increases the risk of osteoporosis, and can increase the risk of premature skin wrinkles. It can increase the risks of the combined contraceptive pill (which is why this type of contraception should not be used in smokers over thirty-five).

Smoking during pregnancy can increase the risk of miscarriage, premature labour and can badly affect the growth of the baby. The health hazards of smoking are directly related to the number of cigarettes (or amount of tobacco) consumed, and also to the tar content. The health risks reduce dramatically once smoking is stopped – so it's never too late to give up. The nicotine in cigarettes is very addictive, which makes giving up incredibly difficult. There is no one method that's universally successful, and it's vital to be completely committed. Some people do manage to successfully give up by gradually cutting down, others just stop completely. Some find nicotine skin patches or gum helpful in reducing cigarette craving, others find hypnosis or acupuncture helpful.

If you've tried and failed to give up successfully on your own, then see your GP, who may be able to refer you to a specialist centre for either counselling or group therapy with others in a similar condition.

STRESS

Everyone needs to have a little stimulation in their day-to-day living – without it, life could become very dull. But for today's women, who is often struggling to run a home, look after the family and earn a living, the stimulation levels can easily become too high. That's stress, and it's bad for your health. Stress can affect every single part of your body.

Symptoms can include:
➤ constantly feeling 'on edge', with a foul temper on a short fuse
➤ sleeping problems
➤ forgetfulness
➤ depression and tearfulness.

But stress doesn't just affect your moods. It can also cause:
➤ headaches and migraines
➤ palpitations and sweating
➤ digestive problems, such as indigestion, bloating, and irritable bowel syndrome (IBS)
➤ teeth grinding
➤ aching joints and muscles
➤ an increase in all the symptoms of PMS.

Worse still, stress can contribute to serious illnesses, such as high blood pressure, heart disease and strokes, and can trigger asthma attacks, eczema and psoriasis.

Self-help
It may be impossible to remove the all sources of stress from your life, but by making a few adjustments you really can reduce your stress load.
➤ Don't try to do too many jobs at once. Sit down for five minutes and write down the chores you feel you need to do, in order of priority. Tackle the most important tasks at the top, but forget about the ones at the bottom unless you really do have time to spare.
➤ Don't try to be a perfectionist, either at home or at work. It really doesn't matter if the kitchen floor isn't spotless. Chances are, no-one will notice anyway, except you!
➤ Learn to delegate, and give away tasks to other people, including the kids. You really don't have to do everything yourself!
➤ Learn to manage your time. Rushing about and doing jobs badly, or leaving them half-finished will only add to your stress levels. Slow down, and try and finish tasks properly, one by one.
➤ Cut down on caffeine (too much can make you irritable), and avoid smoking or drinking too much. Don't skip meals, or grab snacks on the move. Try and sit down to eat three times a day, even if it's only for ten minutes.
➤ Take regular exercise. It can be a great way of releasing pent-up feelings, and relaxing tense muscles.
➤ Make sure you have at least half an hour of relaxation time each day. This can be having a gossip with friends, reading a book, or even just watching the telly (as long as it's not a horror movie!). If you find you really can't sit still, try a relaxation tape. You can buy them from good book or record shops, or may be able to borrow one from your GP.
➤ Some alternative therapies, such as aromatherapy, massage or acupuncture can be helpful.

➤ Bottling up your problems can make them seem worse than they really are. Talk them through with either a good friend or relative who you can trust.

Help from your doctor
If self-help measures don't seem to help you, then do see your GP, but don't expect an instant cure with tranquillizer tablets. A course of counselling or psychotherapy, which your doctor can arrange, will be far more helpful in assisting you to understand and cope with your stress.

SWEATING
Sweating is a vital part of body temperature control. As it evaporates it cools the skin quite effectively, which is why sweating automatically increases in hot weather. On it's own, sweat has no smell – it's only when it mixes with the bacteria that live on the skin's surface that it acquires it's characteristic odour. Some women do sweat more than others, and it can be a cosmetic nuisance.

Self-help for excess sweating
➤ Deodorants only hide the smell of sweat. Always wear an antiperspirant, which actually reduces sweat production. Products containing aluminum chloride (available from chemists) are the most effective.
➤ Avoid synthetic clothes and underwear. Wear clothes made from 100 percent natural fibres instead, such as cotton. These allow sweat to evaporate more easily.
➤ Avoid tight-fitting clothes that cling to your skin.
➤ Wear leather shoes (with leather linings) in the winter. In the summer wear leather sandals, again with a leather insole. Synthetic fibres do not allow your feet to breathe, thus increasing the sweat problem.

Help from your doctor
In very severe cases, surgically dividing the nerves that supply the sweat glands can be effective at reducing sweating.

S

T

TAMPONS

Women of all ages can use tampons, including girls whose periods have only just begun. Young girls and teenagers do, however, often find it painful using hard tampon applicators. Special small non-applicator tampons are now available, and easier for virgins to insert.

Tampons should not be used after childbirth, after an abortion, if you have a vaginal discharge or after any form of vaginal surgery. They should also never be left in for more than six hours at a time, because of the very slight risk of toxic shock syndrome (see page 168). This means that it's best to avoid using tampons overnight, use an external towel instead.

If you think you have lost a tampon inside your vagina, always see a doctor as soon as possible.

THRUSH

Thrush is an infection caused by the yeast candida. It's a common infection in women, affecting mainly the vagina and surrounding genital area, but it can also occasionally occur in the mouth, and around the nipples of breast-feeding mothers.

The main symptoms of genital thrush are soreness and itching, which are usually worse after sex. There is also usually (but not always) a thick creamy vaginal discharge, which has a musty smell. The whole of the genital area can become very red and swollen.

Like all yeasts, thrush thrives in warm, moist conditions. A tiny amount of candida is usually found inside the vagina of most women, but its growth is kept in check by the natural protective acid secretions.

At certain times, however, the conditions in the vagina change, allowing thrush to thrive. These include:
➤ wearing tight-fitting synthetic underwear, which traps sweat and makes the vulval area more moist than normal
➤ reduced acidity due to changing hormone levels. This is why some women are more prone to thrush just before a period, and

why thrush infections are so common during pregnancy. Some women also find that the contraceptive pill makes them more prone to thrush
➤ some antibiotics destroy the protective bacteria, or lactobacilli, that are normally found inside the vagina. This is why a course of penicillin for a sore throat can cause a sore vagina!
➤ an increase in the blood sugar level, particularly when this leads to sugar leaking into the urine. This is why diabetics are more prone to thrush.

Self-help
Very effective treatments for thrush can now be bought directly from chemists. It's important to always treat the inside of the vagina as well as the outside vulval area.
Treatments available include:
➤ anti-fungal creams, such as Canesten and Daktarin
➤ vaginal creams and pessaries, such as Canesten
➤ a single capsule that's taken by mouth, which clears the infection from within, such as Diflucan. This is more expensive, but less messy than using pessaries
➤ alternatively, tea tree oil or pessaries may help to clear mild attacks. Apply two drops of the oil to a damp tampon, and insert into the vagina for two hours. It's best to check yourself for sensitivity to the oil beforehand, by applying a couple of drops to your wrist and waiting for a few hours to ensure no allergic reaction.

Help from your doctor
If you're not sure you have thrush, or if the treatment you have used hasn't helped, then it's important to see your doctor. A swab test will confirm whether your symptoms are due to thrush or another type of infection that requires completely different treatment. Your doctor can also prescribe a wide range of anti-fungal treatments that are only available on prescription.

Prevention
Many women suffer from recurrent attacks of vaginal thrush. These can often be prevented by:
➤ always wearing cotton underwear, which allows sweat to evaporate and helps to prevent a build-up of moisture. Avoid wearing tights (wear stockings instead), and lycra leggings
➤ avoiding douching, as this washes away the protective vaginal secretions

➤ avoiding perfumed bubble baths and soaps, as these can irritate the delicate vaginal skin

➤ boosting the protective bacterial levels by putting natural live yogurt inside the vagina – it's rich in lactobacilli. The easiest way to do this is to dip a non-applicator tampon in the yogurt, then place it inside the vagina for a few hours

➤ using special acid gels (such as Aci-jel, available from chemists) inside the vagina, especially at times when infection is more likely, such as just before a period

Occasionally thrush is passed during sex to men. They get a red itchy rash on the tip of the penis, together with a white discharge that collects under the foreskin. This can be treated very easily with standard anti-fungal creams, but it's important to avoid having sex until both of you are clear of the infection.

THYROID PROBLEMS

The thyroid is a small gland that sits in front of the windpipe in the neck. Its function is to produce the two thyroid hormones, thyroxine (T4) and tri-iodothyronine (T3) which have a powerful effect on the body's metabolism. They also have effects on growth and mental development.

Activity in the thyroid gland is strongly influenced by the thyroid stimulating hormone, (TSH) produced in the pituitary gland at the base of the brain.

Iodine is necessary for the production of this hormone. Adequate amounts can normally be supplied by using table salt that contains iodine. Occasionally iodine deficiency does occur, leading in turn to low levels of thyroid hormone. Iodine deficiency is also one of the conditions that can lead to swelling of the thyroid gland, known as a goitre. If you have a tendency to high blood pressure or water retention then eat seaweed or take kelp supplements (both rich in iodine) instead of salt.

Thyroid gland disorders are ten times more common in women than men and the tendency can run in families.

HYPOTHYROIDISM

This is the medical term for an underactive thyroid. Also known as myxoedema, it can occur at all ages, but is particularly common in older women. Symptoms include chronic tiredness, lethargy, depression, constipation, feeling cold all the time and weight gain. It can also cause dry, thin hair, a dry complexion and erratic, heavy periods. However, it must be said that overall, myxoedema is a rare cause of either chronic tiredness or weight problems!

Left untreated, hypothyroidism can increase the blood cholesterol level, and increase the risk of coronary heart disease. In severe cases, it can also cause quite severe mental changes, with marked slowing down of all mental processes, and eventually it can lead to a coma (although this is rare).

Hypothyroidism can be easily diagnosed by a simple blood test. Treatment is usually straightforward, with replacement thyroid hormone (thyroxine tablets).

HYPERTHYROIDISM
This is the medical term for an overactive thyroid. It's usually caused by a defect of the body's own immune system, which produces an antibody (known as an auto-antibody) that stimulates the thyroid gland into overactivity. In some cases, the auto-antibodies damage the thyroid glandular tissue, and eventually this leads to hypothyroidism.

Symptoms of an overactive thyroid are weight loss, despite a good appetite, sweating, trembling and palpitations. Other symptoms include a dislike of hot weather, frequent bowel motions, general overactivity and being unable to relax. Occasionally, the auto-antibodies associated with hyperthyroidism cause swelling of the tissues behind the eyes, making them protrude with an excessive amount of the white visible.

Diagnosis is again by a simple blood test, which can reveal not only high levels of thyroid hormones, but also high levels of thyroid auto-antibodies.

The drug carbimazole can block the production of thyroid hormone, and may be all the treatment that's required. Beta-blockers, such as propranolol, can help to stop tremors and palpitations. In some cases, it's necessary to remove part or all of the thyroid gland. If the whole gland is removed, thyroid hormone tablets must be given for life to prevent hypothyroidism.

TIREDNESS
Both physical and mental problems can cause tiredness. The most common reason for feeling tired is simply lack of sleep, but this is not as straightforward as it sounds. People vary enormously in the amount of sleep they need, and while some women can survive, and even thrive on as little as five hours a night, others need at least

eight hours to function at their best. Other mental reasons for chronic tiredness include anxiety, stress and depression. All of these can cause disrupted sleep which only adds to the problem.

Any illness can cause tiredness, even a cold or the 'flu. More specifically, tiredness is a common symtom of anaemia, an underactive thyroid gland, and diabetes.

Self-help
➤ Check your sleeping pattern. Put a stop to the late nights, and make a real effort to have at least a week of early nights, so that you can get at least eight hours a sleep a night. It really can make a difference.
➤ Take regular exercise. It will help to increase your energy levels, but also help you to sleep better at night.
➤ Check your diet. Shortage of vital vitamins and minerals can cause tiredness. Don't skip meals, particularly breakfast, and concentrate on eating plenty of foods that give long-lasting energy, such as wholemeal bread, pasta and rice.
➤ Take steps to reduce your anxiety and stress levels (see page 161).

Help from your doctor
➤ Blood tests can check accurately for anaemia, thyroid problems and diabetes.
➤ Anxiety and stress can often be helped by counselling.
➤ Tiredness due to depression can often be quickly relieved with anti-depressant tablets.

TOXIC SHOCK SYNDROME (TSS)

This is an incredibly rare infection that only affects twenty people each year in the UK. It only gets a mention here because about half the cases are linked to using high-absorbency tampons.

TSS is caused by the toxin from certain strains of the bacteria Staphylococcus aureus. Symptoms include a high fever of 40°C or above, muscle pains, vaginal inflammation, vomiting and diarrhoea. Later, a red scaly rash appears, and the person becomes mentally confused.

Anyone with suspected TSS needs urgent medical investigations, and if the diagnosis is confirmed, intensive treatment in hospital.

Anyone who uses tampons should be careful to change them at least once every six hours, and to ensure the last one has been removed at the end of each period.

TOXOPLASMOSIS

This is a disease transmitted to humans by animals. It is usually a fairly minor illness, which produces only mild flu-like symptoms, although occasionally more serious symptoms, such as inflammation in the back of the eye, may occur. However, infection in pregnancy, particularly in the early stages, can have devastating effects on the growing foetus. It can cause miscarriage or stillbirth, or if the baby survives it can cause mental retardation, blindness, enlargement of the liver and brain swelling. Infection can occur either from eating undercooked pork or lamb, or it can be due to inadequate hygiene after handling cat litter (the organism can be excreted in cat faeces). All pregnant women should try and avoid dealing with cat litter. If it's unavoidable, then wash your hands very thoroughly immediately afterwards, and certainly before handling food.

TRICHOMONAS VAGINALIS (TV)

Also known as TV, this is a fairly common sexually transmitted vaginal infection. It's caused by a small amoeba-like organism. In some women the organism can infect the vagina silently for years, but more commonly the infection causes a profuse yellowy green vaginal discharge, with vaginal soreness and itching. Inserting tampons or having intercourse is often very painful.

In men, the infection can cause discomfort and a slight discharge from the urethra (the urine pipe in the penis), but there may be no symptoms at all. The infection can be diagnosed by a simple swab test, which your GP can do. Occasionally the infection is also detected unexpectedly on a cervical smear test. Treatment is with the antibiotic metronidazole, either as a very large single dose, or as a course over five days. All women diagnosed with trichomonas should have thorough tests to check for other sexually transmitted infections, such as gonorrhoea. Sexual partners should always have treatment at the same time, to prevent reinfection.

TUBAL PREGNANCY

(see Ectopic Preganancy page 60).

T

U

ULTRASOUND

This is a diagnostic technique that uses reflected sound waves of a very high frequency to give a picture of the internal organs of the body. Although it was used mainly in gynaecology and maternity care, it's now increasingly used to investigate other parts of the body, such as the heart, gallbladder, breasts and kidneys. Unlike X-rays, which involve a tiny amount of radiation, ultrasound is considered to be safe and harmless.

Ultrasound can only be used to investigate structures that are either soft, or filled with fluid. The sound waves don't pass through gas or bone, so it can't be used to look at the brain (which is surrounded by bone) or the lungs or intestines (which are full of gas).

A small probe is used, which is gently moved across the area being examined. An ultrasound of the pelvic organs is traditionally done with the probe on the surface of the lower abdomen, but more detailed images can be obtained using a special probe placed inside the vagina – special sheaths are used over the probe to prevent any infection passing between patients!

URINARY PROBLEMS

(see Incontinence page 103 and Cystitis page 46.)

UTERUS

This is the proper medical name for the womb. It's a small pear-shaped structure, normally between 8.5–10cm in length, weighing 60–90g. It has a central hollow cavity that is surrounded by thick, muscular walls. The lower part of the womb narrows to form a long neck, or cervix. A small passageway leads out through the cervix and into the vagina. The Fallopian tubes attach at the top of the womb on each side.

The womb develops from two halves, which normally fuse in the midline. In about 1 percent of women, there is an abnormality of the womb, usually as a result of a fusion error. This can be anything from just a small septum inside the womb, to two completely separate wombs, each with its own cervix and upper vagina.

During pregnancy, the womb muscle increases enormously to accommodate the growing baby, and just before the baby is born the womb weighs about 1kg. Afterwards, it shrinks dramatically, but tends to remain slightly larger than before the pregnancy. After the menopause the womb becomes much smaller than before pregnancy.

Special tissue, the endometrium, lines the womb cavity. This changes in response to hormones produced by the ovaries, and is shed as a period approximately once a month. The womb itself does not produce any hormones at all – it's only real function is to act as an incubator for babies!

In 70 percent of women, the womb lies tilted forwards in the pelvis. In the remaining 30 percent, it's retroverted, or tilted backwards. This is nothing to worry about, and does not usually cause any symptoms, though period pains in these women may be felt more in the back than in others.

UTERINE FIBROIDS

These are balls of muscle that develop within the wall of the womb. They are usually quite small (and may only be the size of a pea) but they can grow very large (to the size of a grapefruit). There may be just one, or several of them.

They are present in at least 20 percent of women over thirty. In many cases, they do not produce any symptoms, and the women are unaware that they are there. However, if they distort the lining of the womb they can cause heavy and prolonged periods, and if they are large they can cause pelvic discomfort. They can also put pressure on the bladder, leading to a need to pass urine frequently. Less often, large fibroids can press backwards, causing backache. Large fibroids, particularly ones that distort the cavity of the womb, can cause infertility and repeated miscarriages.

Exactly why some women develop fibroids and others don't is a mystery, but the hormone oestrogen does stimulate their growth. They commonly appear after a pregnancy, and shrink after the menopause, when oestrogen levels fall.They can often be detected during a routine pelvic examination. An ultrasound scan can give a more detailed picture of their size and position.

Fibroids that are not causing any symptoms can be safely left alone. They do not turn cancerous. Larger fibroids can be shrunk using drugs that reduce oestrogen levels, such as Zoladex. However,

U

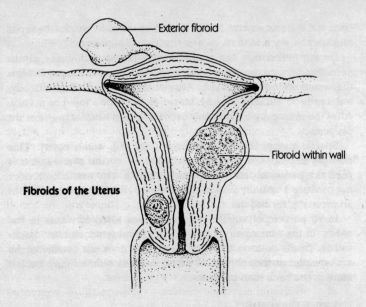

Exterior fibroid

Fibroid within wall

Fibroids of the Uterus

this is only a short-term cure, and the best treatment for very troublesome fibroids is to have them removed.

Occasionally it's possible to remove just the fibroids (a myomectomy), but a hysterectomy is often required, especially if there are multiple fibroids present. Fibroids are not dangerous, so the decision to go ahead with this type of operation must be based on the severity of the symptoms they are causing.

CANCER OF THE UTERUS

There are two types of uterine cancer – cancer of the neck of the womb, or cervix (see page 37) and cancer of the womb lining (endometrial cancer). This is slightly less common than cervical cancer, but still more than 3,500 women are newly affected each year.

Some women are more at risk than others of developing endometrial cancer. These include

➤ women who have had no children
➤ women who are overweight
➤ women who have taken oestrogen-only hormone-replacement therapy (HRT), without added progesterone.

However, taking the combined contraceptive pill can help to protect against endometrial (and ovarian) cancer. Though endometrial cancer can occur at any age, it is most common in women between the ages of fifty and seventy. The first sign is abnormal bleeding – in younger women this can be heavy, prolonged periods, or erratic bleeding in-between periods. In post-menopausal women the first sign is often a blood stained vaginal discharge. This is why any vaginal bleeding that occurs after the menopause should be investigated promptly by a doctor. In some cases, particularly when the bleeding is light, inflamed and dry vaginal walls are to blame, but it's essential that a pelvic ultrasound (see page 170), and a biopsy of the womb lining are done to rule out cancer. A cervical smear test only checks for cervical cancer – it is not a test for endometrial cancer.

Treatment usually involves removing the whole womb, the Fallopian tubes and the ovaries, together sometimes with the lymph nodes from the pelvis. Follow-up treatment with radiotherapy and chemotherapy may be required if there is evidence that the cancer cells may have spread from the womb. Overall, treatment for endometrial cancer is very effective, and more than 80 percent of sufferers are still alive more than five years later.

For information on period problems see page 136. For information on womb prolapse, see page 146.

U

V

THE VAGINA

The vagina is a muscular tube, approximately 6in (15cm) in length along its back wall. The walls are usually covered in moist secretions from the lining, that contain numerous healthy bacteria, known as lactobacilli. Around the time of ovulation, and during sexual excitement, there's usually a noticeable increase in these natural secretions.

Just inside the vagina entrance is a thin membrane, the hymen. In virgins, this has a small opening, which allows the passage of

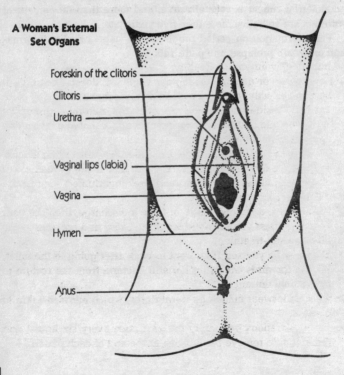

A Woman's External Sex Organs

Foreskin of the clitoris

Clitoris

Urethra

Vaginal lips (labia)

Vagina

Hymen

Anus

menstrual blood. When a woman first has sex the hymen has to stretch, or more usually tear slightly, to allow the penis to enter the vagina. Some (but not all) women find this slightly painful, and it may also cause slight bleeding.

After the menopause, the lining of the vagina becomes much more dry, thin and fragile, and this can cause slight pain and bleeding on intercourse. This problem can be eased by using a lubricating jelly, and in the more long term, by the use of hormone-replacement therapy (HRT) or vaginal oestrogen cream.

Vaginal itching has two main causes. The most common is irritation from chemicals, such as perfumed soaps, bubble baths, and vaginal deodorants. An infection may also be to blame, particularly thrush (see page 164) and trichomonas vaginalis (see page 169).

Vaginal soreness can also be due to irritation, but is more likely to be due to an infection. (See page 156 for more information, and advice about vaginal discharge. The section on painful sex [see page 154] gives more information about vaginal problems during sex.)

Self-help
To help keep your vagina healthy:
➤ never wash or douche inside your vagina. It doesn't need it – it has a perfectly good self-cleansing mechanism of its own! Washing inside the vagina removes the naturally protective secretions and, apart from causing irritation, can make the vagina more susceptible to infections
➤ avoid using chemicals, such as antiseptics, including Dettol, soaps and bubble baths around the entrance to the vagina. Avoid all bath additives if possible, and use unperfumed soap in the vulval area
➤ if you notice a strange smell, or have a discharge, then see your doctor – unless you're confident of the cause and are able to use effective self-treatment
➤ always wipe yourself from front to back after going to the toilet. Wiping forwards can bring harmful bacteria from the rectum to the vaginal entrance
➤ wear underwear made of natural fibres, which allow the skin to breathe
➤ change tampons frequently (at least once every six hours) and remember to remove the last one at the end of each period.

V

VARICOSE VEINS

Large, twisted and swollen veins can occur anywhere on the body, but the area most frequently affected is the back of the legs.

At least a quarter of all women will get varicose veins – that's double the rate for men. Inside the leg veins are numerous small valves that act as tiny dams and prevent blood flowing backwards down the legs with gravity. Any weakening of these valves leads to pooling of blood in the vein below. This vein eventually becomes stretched and distorted – a varicose vein.

Varicose veins often develop during pregnancy, as a result of the increased pressure on the pelvic veins from the heavy growing womb. They're also more common in women who are overweight (due to a similar 'back pressure' effect) and in women who spend hours on their feet. They also tend to run in families.

Varicose veins can vary between very large, obvious blue ropes, and tiny red or blue threads, visible just beneath the skin (often on the thighs). Though small veins tend to be just a cosmetic problem, larger veins can ache, and lead to swollen ankles at the end of the day. Left untreated for years they can also increase the risk of leg ulcers, and occasionally become inflamed – a condition known as phlebitis. Women with large varicose veins are also slightly more at risk of having a deep vein thrombosis, and they should avoid taking the combined oral contraceptive pill if possible.

Self-help
You can help to prevent and ease varicose veins by:
➤ keeping to a normal weight for your height
➤ keeping active and taking regular exercise. Swimming, cycling and walking are particularly good for legs
➤ avoiding long periods of standing. If you are on your feet for hours on end, wear support tights
➤ sitting with your feet up when you can
➤ avoid wearing clothes that are very tight around the upper thigh or waist, such as girdles, and avoiding tight pop socks which can constrict the blood flow up your calves
➤ wearing support tights during pregnancy, especially if you have a family history of varicose veins.

Help from your doctor
Small spider veins can be treated by either sclerotherapy (when a special sealing chemical is injected into the veins) or by laser

surgery. As this is usually a cosmetic procedure, it's rarely available on the NHS.

Larger veins are usually treated by surgical removal. If only a few veins in the lower leg are affected, these alone can be removed through a series of tiny cuts. Larger veins can be removed in their entirety using a wire that's inserted into the vein in the groin. Though this usually only involves a one day stay in hospital, it's important to wear strong support stockings for several weeks afterwards.

VITAMINS AND MINERALS

Vitamins and minerals are naturally occurring substances that are essential for the body to function normally. Although only tiny amounts of each are required, any shortage can cause severe health problems.

There is increasing debate amongst the medical profession about the amounts of vitamins that are needed for good health. There are two basic groups of vitamins: Vitamins A, D, E and K are fat soluble, and excess amounts can be stored in the liver and used if necessary by the body over a period of six months. The B vitamins and vitamin C are soluble in water, and can't be stored in the body. Any excess is passed out of the body immediately in the urine.

For each vitamin there is a recommended daily allowance, or RDA, that is the amount required by the average person to maintain good health. The values in the table are those set by the European Community in 1993. Although these can be useful as a general guide to see if you are likely to be going short of any individual vitamin, there is increasing evidence that eating more than the RDA for some vitamins can be beneficial to good health. This applies particularly to the antioxidant vitamins C, E and beta-carotene (a form of vitamin A). These vitamins mop up harmful chemicals (known as free radicals) in the body tissues, and can help to prevent heart disease and some cancers. However, eating large amounts of other vitamins, particularly some of the B vitamins, can be harmful and large doses of vitamin A can be dangerous in pregnancy.

A healthy, well-balanced diet, with plenty of fresh fruit and vegetables, should provide all the vitamins and minerals that a normal women needs for good health. However, some women may have higher requirements. Smokers need more vitamin C, chromium and zinc, and women on the combined contraceptive pill may benefit from taking additional vitamin B6 and folic acid. Older women at risk of osteoporosis may also benefit from taking

V

additional vitamin D, as this aids absorption of calcium, which is essential for strong bones.

However, taking large amounts of most vitamins can be harmful, and taking mega doses can be downright dangerous. For instance, high doses of vitamin A in pregnancy can damage the growing baby. Don't be fooled into thinking that swallowing handfuls of supplements each morning is going to make you super healthy – it may have the exactly the opposite effect. Good looks and good health are more likely to come from a healthy diet, plenty of exercise and relaxation than from a bottle of pills.

VITAMIN CHART – SEE OVERLEAF

VULVAL PROBLEMS

The vulva is the medical name for the external genital area. It includes the skin surrounding the clitoris, and the openings of the bladder and vagina.

Vulval itching and soreness

This can be caused by:
➤ irritation and allergy due to contact with perfumed soaps, bubble baths, talcum powder, vaginal deodorants, and clothes washed in biological washing powder
➤ infections, particularly thrush
➤ skin disorders, such as eczema, psoriasis, and more unusually, lichen sclerosis. This is a condition similar to eczema, that causes itchy, scaly white areas around the vulva. Similar white areas can also be found elsewhere on the body, especially in the mouth
➤ genital warts
➤ genital herpes.

Self-help

If you're prone to itching and soreness, avoid using any bath additives at all, and always use an unperfumed soap. Use non-biological detergents for washing your underwear, and if you use a fabric conditioner, use a brand that's labelled as suitable for sensitive skin. Avoid using any form of 'feminine deodorant' or talc in the vulval area.

Thrush can usually be effectively treated with pessaries and creams available from chemists. Most thrush originates inside the vagina, and using cream alone on the outside won't be effective.

V

Have a look at your vulva using a mirror. If you see any unusual lumps (which could be warts) or any whitened areas of skin, then it's important to see a doctor.

Help from your doctor
Any infection can be accurately diagnosed by a simple swab test. Your doctor can then prescribe appropriate treatment. A specialist dermatologist's opinion is usually required to diagnose and treat skin conditions such as eczema, psoriasis or lichen sclerosis. Occasionally it's also necessary for a tiny biopsy to be taken for a firm diagnosis. Treatment of all of these conditions is usually with steroid creams, of varying strengths.

Occasionally white patches, particularly in older women, are due to abnormal, or precancerous cells. This is why persistent white areas of skin in this area should never be ignored. These are usually treated by surgical excision.

Vulval pain, or vulvodynia
This can be due to numerous conditions, including all of those that cause vulval itching, listed above. However, in some women there is no obvious cause, yet they have persistent pain and discomfort in the vulval area, especially during intercourse. In some women a chronic low-grade infection, with either thrush, herpes or the genital wart virus is to blame, which in turn triggers low-grade inflammation, leading to vulval pain. It can also be due to low-grade inflammation of the vestibular glands, which lie just inside the inner folds of the vulva. Stress, a poor diet, and being overtired can all make vulvodynia worse. Many women with vulval pain are also depressed, and this may contribute to their pain. Treatment with anti-depressant tablets is often helpful, especially when other local treatments fail.

V

Vitamin Chart

VITAMIN	NEEDED FOR	FOUND IN	DEFICIENCY EFFECTS	OVERDOSE EFFECTS	RECOMMENDED DAILY DOSE
A Is found in 2 forms:					
1) Retinol	Healthy skin, teeth and bones, good vision	Liver, fish, eggs, dairy produce	Dry eyes, poor vision, especially at night. Increased risk of skin infections	Enlarged liver and spleen. In pregnancy can cause abnormalities in the baby	800mcg daily, 1,200mcg for breast-feeding mums
2) Beta-carotene	Is an anti-oxidant, and so can help prevent heart disease and some cancers	Carrots, spinach, watercress, broccoli		Beta-carotene appears to be non-toxic	A separate dose for beta-carotene has not been established
B1 (thiamine)	Healthy nerves and muscles, getting energy from foods	Yeast extract, brown rice, dried beans, fortified breakfast cereals	Tiredness, muscle weakness, nausea, loss of appetite	Headache, irritability, weakness, rapid pulse	1.4mg. Athletes, pregnant and breast-feeding mums may need more
B2 (ribo-flavin)	The release of energy from food. Also healthy hair, teeth and nails	Yeast extract, and dairy produce such as milk, eggs and cheese	Sores and cracks around the mouth		1.6mg. Women on the contraceptive pill, heavy smokers and drinkers may need more

V

	Good for	Sources	Deficiency	Excess	Recommended daily amount
B6 (pyridoxine)	Healthy skin, nerves and muscles. Also for the production of antibodies which help the body fight infection	Wholegrain cereals, yeast extract, nuts, and bananas	Anaemia and skin complaints, muscle weakness and irritability. May contribute to PMS	Permanent nerve damage, causing walking difficulties, numbness and tingling	2mg a day. Women taking B6 as a treatment for PMS should take no more than 50mg daily
B12	The formation of healthy red blood cells	Beef, pork, liver, eggs. Also fortified breakfast cereals	Pernicious anaemia, low energy levels		1mcg. Smokers and heavy drinkers may require slightly more. Vegans are at risk of deficiency
Pantothenic acid	Helps the body to release energy from food. Also helps in the formation of antibodies, and some hormones	Yeast extract, liver, eggs, wholemeal flour and dried fruit	Loss of appetite, abdominal pain and some nerve and psychiatric disorders	Nausea, bloating, tiredness and diarrhoea	6mg
Niacin (nico-tinic acid)	Helps to regulate metabolism, and release energy from food	Meat, poultry, oily fish, wholegrain cereals	Fatigue, weakness, loss of appetite, and minor skin problems	Headache, tiredness, and urticarial skin rashes	18mg. Heavy drinkers may need more

V

Vitamin Chart

VITAMIN	NEEDED FOR	FOUND IN	DEFICIENCY EFFECTS	OVERDOSE EFFECTS	RECOMMENDED DAILY DOSE
Folic Acid	The formation of healthy red blood cells. Also helps to prevent spina bifida	Wheatgerm, liver, broccoli, green cabbage and yeast extract	Anaemia and other blood disorders. Deficiency during pregnancy can increase the risk in the baby of spina bifida and other neural tube defects	May mask a vitamin B12 deficiency	200mcg. Women planning a baby should take 400mcg daily, and continue this dose 12 weeks into the pregnancy
C Ascorbic acid	Helps to protect against infections, and also improves resistance against viruses and bacteria. Is also an antioxidant so can help to prevent heart disease and some cancers	Citrus fruits, cabbage, red and green peppers, potatoes and tomatoes	Increased susceptibility to infections and slow healing of wounds. Weakness, irritability, bleeding gums and weight loss	Diarrhoea, kidney stones	60mg. Diabetics, pregnant and breast-feeding mums, and those under severe stress or recovering from an illness may need more. Smokers need 2 to 3 times more, as heavy smoking increases the rate that vitamin C is used by the body

V

D	Healthy bones and teeth. Aids the absorption of calcium from the intestines	Fish, liver, oils, eggs, milk, and fortified margarines. Vitamin D is produced in the skin in strong sunlight	Soft, weak bones, and poor bone formation in children (rickets)	Likely at doses of 10mcg a day or more – nausea and vomiting, kidney stones and kidney failure	5mcg. Pregnant and breast-feeding mums may need slightly more
E	Is a powerful antioxidant, and can help to prevent heart disease. Also promotes healthy skin	Wheatgerm, nuts, especially peanuts, margarine and wholemeal bread	Can lead to anaemia, particularly in babies	Tiredness, diarrhoea, and other digestive disturbances	10mg. Breast-feeding women – 13mg
K	Essential for normal blood clotting	Liver, vegetable oils, milk	Bleeding disorders	Anaemia, nerve problems	65mcg. New-born babies need a supplement of vitamin K soon after birth, to prevent spontaneous bleeding from defective blood clotting

V

IMPORTANT MINERALS

(There are 25 that are needed – these are the 8 main ones)

MINERAL	ESSENTIAL FOR	GOOD SOURCES	DEFICIENCY SYMPTOMS	RDA
Calcium	Strong bones and teeth	Dairy produce, such as milk, cheese, yoghurt. Also canned fish and green leafy vegetables. Vitamin D is essential for absorbing calcium from food	Brittle, fragile bones, and weak teeth	Officially 800mg, but most women would benefit from at least 1000mg daily. Pregnant and breast-feeding mums require 1500mg
Iron	The formation of healthy red blood cells, which carry oxygen in the bloodstream	Red meat and offal, eggs, spinach and raisins. Vitamin C aids iron absorption from food	Anaemia, with tiredness, and lack of energy. Also a sore tongue, and hair loss	14mg a day – more during pregnancy, or if you have heavy periods
Sodium	Healthy cells throughout the body. Together with potassium, sodium controls the amount of fluid in the body, and is important for normal kidney function	Table salt. Also salty foods such as smoked meats, and salted nuts and crisps	Lack of sodium is rare, but can occur in severe dehydration, especially in hot climates. This can cause weakness, thirst, and a fall in blood pressure	1.6g a day. Most people eat at least 50% more than their body needs
Potassium	Healthy cells, and regulation of the fluid balance in the body	Apples, bananas, carrots, broccoli and oranges	Vomiting, diarrhoea, weak muscles and loss of appetite	3.5g a day. People taking diuretics (waterpills) require more

V

184

Mineral Chart

MINERAL	ESSENTIAL FOR	GOOD SOURCES	DEFICIENCY SYMPTOMS	RDA
Magnesium	For release of energy from food. Also for healthy nerves and muscles, and strong bones	Nuts, soya beans, wholemeal flour, dried fruit	Tiredness, dizziness and muscle cramps	300mg a day
Phosphorus	For healthy bones and teeth, and for energy production	Cheddar cheese, canned fish, eggs, yoghurt. 10% of our daily supply usually comes from food additives	Defiency is rare – but can cause weakness, joint stiffness and confusion	800mg a day
Zinc	Vital for proper growth and functioning of whole body. Also for ovulation, fertilization and, in men for the formation of testosterone and mature sperm	Sea foods especially oysters, most meat, wheatgerm and lentils	Increased risk of infections, skin rashes, tiredness and a poor appetite. Lack of zinc has also been linked with increased risk of infertility, miscarriage and prema-ture labour	15mg a day, more in pregnancy and breast-feeding
Selenium	Is an anti-oxidant, and works with vitamins A,C and E to help protect cells from damage from free radicals. Also helps the immune system	Wholewheat foods, liver, kidney, fish and shellfish	Tiredness and lack of energy. Lack of any of the antioxidants may increase the risk of heart disease and some cancers	60mcg a day, more during breast feeding

V

WARTS

Warts are caused by an infection with the human papilloma virus (or HPV). They can occur anywhere on the body, but most commonly affect the hands and feet, where they grow inwards, causing a verruca. The virus can also be passed during sexual contact, leading to genital warts.

Genital warts are important because infection of the cervix with some strains of HPV is probably an important risk factor for developing cervical cancer, and warts in the vagina or vulva may lead later to abnormal cells. All genital warts should be promptly treated, and all women who've had genital warts should have yearly smear tests. Elsewhere on the body, about 50 percent of warts disappear on their own in about six to twelve months, but treatment is advisable if they appear to be spreading, are painful, or if they are cosmetically unsightly. Many can be successfully self-treated or they can be treated by your doctor.

Self-help
This is only advisable for warts on the hands and for verrucas. Never attempt to self-treat those on the genital area or the face.

Various wart paints are available from chemists. Carefully apply the paint to just the wart – if necessary protect the surrounding skin with a plaster. Leave the paint on for twenty-four hours (or less according to the instructions on the bottle), then wash it off. Next, and this is very important, rub off the hardened surface layer vigorously with either a pumice stone or a nail file. Then apply another layer of wart paint, for another twenty-four hours, and so on. With perseverance, most warts and verrucas will clear.

Help from your doctor
Cryotherapy (a form of super-cold freezing) involves spraying the wart with liquid nitrogen. Many GPs, as well as hospital dermatologists, now offer this as a treatment. Alternatively, warts can be destroyed by heat, using cautery or lasers. Genital warts can be treated either by repeated applications of podophyllin paint, or by cryotherapy.

W

WEIGHT PROBLEMS

There are very few women who are happy with their weight – some feel too thin, but many more feel too fat. Images of skinny models mean that many women are striving for a weight that is actually too low. An ideal medical weight is often heavier than many people realize – and it means having a body that's fairly well covered with female curves as nature intended. Doctors calculate ideal weight using a measurement of body mass index (BMI). This is your weight in kilos, divided by the square of your height in metres. For example, a woman weighing 70kg, and 1.69m tall, has a BMI of 24.5 (70÷1.69x1.69=24.5). A BMI of 20–25 means your weight is ideal; those with a BMI under 20 are medically underweight, and are at risk of medical problems such as osteoporosis, irregular or non-existent periods and infertility. Those in the range 25–30 are overweight, and those with a BMI greater than 35 are medically obese, and have a 30 percent increased risk of heart disease, diabetes, high blood pressure, and osteo-arthritis. Check your weight on the chart at the base of the previous page.

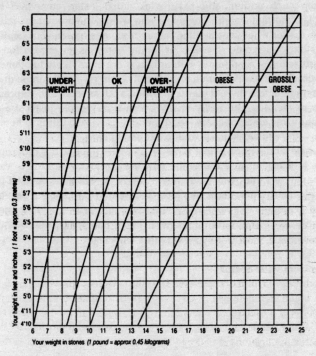

187

W

UNDERWEIGHT

There are some people who stay thin, no matter what they eat, because of a naturally high metabolic rate. Many would regard this as good fortune, but for some skinny people it can be a real problem, especially in the winter when the lack of natural insulation can mean they feel the cold much more than others.

Unintentional weight loss can be caused by a low appetite, often as a result of stress, or depression. It can also be caused by an over-active thyroid gland, diabetes, a digestive problem or more rarely, by an internal cancer. Continued weight loss, when you're not on a diet, should always be investigated by a doctor. Extreme weight loss is also a sign of anorexia nervosa (see page 15).

OVERWEIGHT

Being overweight doesn't just affect your looks – it can affect your health too.

It increases the risk of high blood pressure, strokes, heart disease and diabetes. The extra load on the joints means that osteoarthritis occurs much earlier, and progresses much faster, compared to people of normal weight. The more your weigh, the greater the risk.

No matter what your mother, father or anyone else in your family looks like, it's wrong to use your family genes as an excuse for a weight problem. Bad family eating habits are more likely to blame!

Occasionally, weight gain (or difficulty losing weight) can be due to an underactive thyroid gland, or drugs, such as some anti-depressants or steroids. But sadly, many overweight people just have a naturally low metabolic rate – and the only answer to this is to boost it up with regular exercise, and to eat carefully.

Whole libraries of books have been written about the different ways to slim, but in the end the only way to lose weight is to eat fewer calories than your body needs. Body fat will then be used to provide energy. You can make a big difference to the second part of the equation – the amount of energy you need – by exercise. Exercise not only burns up calories, but it also boosts the body's metabolism for some time afterwards. The more often, and more vigorously you exercise, the greater the effect!

For more information on slimming pills, see page 159.

WOMB

(see Uterus page 170.)

Useful Addresses

Alcoholics Anonymous
PO Box 1,
Stonebow House,
Stonebow,
York YO1 2NJ
01904 644 026
*Mutual support and guidance
for those with an alcohol
problem.*

Alanon Family Groups
61 Great Dover St,
London SE1 4YF
0171 403 0888
*Support for families and friends
of alcoholics.*

**Arthritis and Rheumatism
Council for Research**
Copeman House,
St Mary's Court,
St Mary's Gate,
Chesterfield S41 7TD
*Information on rheumatic
diseases and arthritis, including
joint replacements.*

**Association of Continence
Advice**
The Basement,
2 Doughty St,
London WC1N 2PH
0171 404 6875
*Information and advice about
incontinence.*

**BACUP – British Association of
Cancer United Patients**
3 Bath Place,
Rivington St,
London EC2A 3JR
0171 613 2121
*Information, practical advice
and support for cancer patients,
their families and friends.*

Breast Cancer Care
15–19 Britten St,
London SW3 3TZ
01500 245 345
*Advice and support for women
with breast cancer.*

**British Acupuncture
Association and Register**
34 Alderney St,
London SW1V 4EU
*List of registered acupuncturists
available.*

**British Association of Aesthetic
and Plastic Surgeons (BAAPS)**
Royal College of Surgeons,
35–43 Lincoln's Inn Fields,
London WC2A 3PN
0171 636 4864
*Advice about plastic surgery
procedures, and list of
accredited surgeons.*

British Association of Counselling
1 Regent Place,
Rugby,
Worcs CV21 2PJ
List of qualified practitioners, and advice about low-cost schemes for counselling.

British Association for Sexual and Marital Therapy
PO Box 63,
Sheffield,
S. Yorks S10 3TS
List of qualified practitioners.

British Heart Foundation
14 Fitzharding St,
London W1H 4DH
0171 935 0185
Wide range of information leaflets about all aspects of heart disease.

British Homoepathic Association
27A Devonshire St,
London W1N 1RJ
0171 935 2163
List of practitioners, plus information about homeopathy.

British Migraine Association
178A High Rd,
Byfleet,
West Byfleet,
Surrey. KT14 7ED
Information and support for sufferers.

Cruse – Bereavement Care
Cruse House,
126 Sheen Rd,
Richmond,
Surrey TW9 1UR
0181 940 4818
Counselling and practical advice for anyone who has been bereaved.

Eating Disorders Association
Sackville Place,
44 Magdalen St,
Norwich NR3 1JU
01603 621 414
Information and support for those suffering from anorexia and bulimia.

Gingerbread
49 Wellington St,
London WC2E 7BN
0171 240 0953
Self-help association for one parent families.

Hairline International
Lyons Court,
1668 High St,
Knowle,
West Midlands
01564 775 281
Information and advice for people who, for any reason, lose their hair.

Herpes Association
41 North Rd,
London, N7 9DP
0171 609 9061
Information and advice about herpes and shingles.

Impotence Information Centre
PO Box 1130,
London W3 0BB
Information about impotence.

Issue – National Fertility Association
509 Aldridge Rd,
Great Barr,
Birmingham B44 8NA
0121 344 4414
Information and advice for people with fertility problems.

ME Association
Stanhope House,
High St,
Stamford-le-Hope,
Essex. SS17 OHA
01375 361 013
Information and advice about ME.

Miscarriage Association
c/o Clayton Hospital,
Northgate,
Wakefield,
West Yorkshire WF1 3JS
01924 200 799
Support and advice for those who have a miscarriage.

National Association for Premenstrual Syndrome
PO Box 72,
Sevenoaks,
Kent TN13 1XQ
01732 741 709
Information and advice about premenstrual syndrome.

National Eczema Society
4 Tavistock Pl,
London WC1H 9RA
0171 388 4097
Support and advice for eczema sufferers and their families.

National Endometriosis Society
35 Belgrave Sq,
London SW1X 8QB
0171 235 4137
Information and advice about endometriosis.

National Osteoporosis Society
PO Box 10,
Radstock,
Bath BA3 3YB
01761 432 472
Information and advice about osteoporosis.

Pelvic Inflammatory Disease Network
52 Featherstone St,
London EC1Y 8RT
0171 251 6580
Information and advice about PID.

Positively Women
347–9 City Road,
London EC1V 1LR
0171 713 0444
Support group for HIV-Positive women.

Psoriasis Association
7 Milton St,
Northampton NN2 7JG
01604 711 129
Information and advice about psoriasis.

Quitline
Victory House,
170 Tottenham Court Rd,
London W1P 0HA
0171 487 3000
Help and information for those
who want to stop smoking.

Rape Crisis Centre
PO Box 69,
London, WCLX 9NJ
0171 837 1600
Twenty-four-hour counselling,
medical and legal help for
victims.

Relate – National Marriage
Guidance
Herbert Gray College,
Little Church St,
Rugby,
Warks CV21 3AP
01788 573 241

Resolve – The Vaginismus
Support Group
PO Box 820,
London, N10 3AW
Information for sufferers, who
can then contact one another.

Royal College of Surgeons
35–43 Lincolns Inn Fields,
London WC2A 7PN
0171 405 3474

The Samaritans
10 The Grove,
Slough,
Berks SL1 1QP
01753 532 713
Local numbers are listed in the
telephone directory. *Support for*
all those in distress. 184
branches open 24 hours a day.

Seasonal Affective Disorder
Association
PO Box 989,
London, SW7 2PZ
0181 969 7028
Help and information for
sufferers.

Victim Support
Cranmer House,
39 Brixton Rd,
London, SW9 6DZ
0171 735 9166
Offers practical information,
advice and emotional support
for victims of crime.

Womens Aid Federation
for England
PO Box 391,
Bristol BS99 7WS
0345 023468
Advice, information and
support for abused women.

Womens Health Concern
83 Earls Court Rd,
London, W8 6EF
0171 938 3932
Advice for women with
gynaecological and other
health problems.